Long-Term Care in Transition
THE REGULATION OF NURSING HOMES

Long-Term Care in Transition

THE REGULATION OF NURSING HOMES

David Barton Smith

AUPHA Press

Library of Congress Cataloging in Publication Data

Smith, David Barton.
    Long-term care in transition.

    Bibliography: p.
    Includes index.
    1. Nursing homes—Law and legislation—United
States. 2. Nursing homes—Law and legislation—New
York (State) I. Title. [DNLM: 1. Long term care—
United States—Legislation. 2. Nursing homes—United
States—Legislation. WX 32 AA1 S6L]
KF3826.N8S63   344.73'03216   81-72
ISBN 0-914904-65-5

The study described in this book was supported by a
grant from the National Center for Health Services Research, Office of Health Policy, Research and Statistics,
Department of Health and Human Services Grant number 1 ROI HS 02694-01.

AUPHA Press is an imprint of Health Administration Press.
Health Administration Press   AUPHA Press
School of Public Health   One DuPont Circle
The University of Michigan   Washington, D.C. 20036
Ann Arbor, Michigan 48109
        313-764-1380   202-659-4354

"I'm just a working stiff,
I'm not a crusader,
I'm only doing my job."

This book is dedicated to those working in the health sector who, in spite of the immense difficulties and personal sacrifices, and with sometimes awesome, quiet courage, do just that.

Contents

List of Figures viii

List of Tables x

Acknowledgements xii

Preface xiv

Chapter One   Nursing Homes on the Cutting Edge 1

Emergence of Professional Controls 1

Emergence of Public Regulation 6

Emerging Contradictions in Control 10

New York State's Regulatory Offensive 13

Chapter Two   Tightening Professional Controls 19

Regulatory Changes 25

Legislative Initiatives 25

Administrative Initiatives 25

Results 26

Restricting Entry 26

Enforcing Standards 33

Conclusions 52

Chapter Three   Tightening Fiscal Controls 56

Changes 66

Administrative Changes 66

Legislative Reforms 66

Changes in Capital Cost Reimbursement 68

Cost Control 69

Relating Reimbursement to Quality of Care 69

Summary of Changes 70

Results   71
    Control of Abuse   71
    Control of Costs   74
    Linking Reimbursement to Quality of Care   78
Conclusions   84

Chapter Four   Strengthening Criminal Enforcement   91

Background   91
Convictions   99
Recouping Fraudulent Medicaid Payments   104
Patient Abuse   112
Public Misconduct   113
Conclusions   120

Chapter Five   Enhancing Consumer Controls   126

Changes   129
    Disseminating Information to Consumers and
        Their Families   130
    Making Standards More Responsive to Consumers   130
    Improving Consumer Access to the Redress
        of Grievances   131
    Enhancing the Psychological and Legal Senses
        of Ownership   132
Results of Disseminating Information   133
Results of More Responsive Standards   134
Results of Improving Access to Redress   135
Results of Enhancing the Sense of Ownership   142
Conclusions   146

Chapter Six   Summary and Conclusions   148

Results   149
    Professional Standards and Surveillance   149
    Reimbursement   149
    Criminal Enforcement   150
    Consumer Control   150
Remaining Questions   150
Prescriptions   153

References   157
Index   164

List of Figures

Figure 1.1 Increase in Number of Nursing Home Beds in
New York State, 1964–79   12

Figure 1.2 Number of Articles Indexed in *The New York
Times* Under the Heading "Nursing
Homes," 1956–78   14

Figure 2.1 Disciplinary Action Taken Against Nursing
Home Administrators by the New York
State Board of Examiners   31

Figure 2.2 Reported Number of Revocations of License
and Disciplinary Actions for Physicians in
the United States, 1962–78   32

Figure 2.3 Openings and Closings of Skilled Nursing
Facilities in New York State by Number of
Facilities, 1966–78   37

Figure 2.4 Openings and Closings of Skilled Nursing
Facilities in New York State by Number of
Beds Gained or Lost, 1966–78   38

Figure 2.5 Openings and Closings of Skilled Nursing
Facilities in New York State by Percent
Proprietary Ownership, 1966–78   39

Figure 2.6 Openings and Closings of Skilled Nursing
Facilities in New York State by Average
Number of Beds, 1966–78   40

Figure 2.7 Proposed Review Process for Long-Term Care
Facilities   51

Figure 2.8 The Ebb and Flow of Health Care Standards
Regulation   54

Figure 3.1 Increase in Number of Nursing Home Beds in New York State by Ownership, 1930–74 58

Figure 3.2 Calculation of Medicaid Reimbursement Rate as of January 1, 1975 63

Figure 3.3 Organizational Chart of the New York State Department of Health 67

Figure 3.4 New York State Medicaid Payments from Fiscal Year 1966–67 to Fiscal Year 1978–79 75

Figure 3.5 New York State Medicaid Payments for Nursing Home Care from Fiscal Year 1966–67 to Fiscal Year 1978–79, by Percent Increase 89

Figure 4.1 *New York Times* Articles Dealing with Criminal Aspects of the Nursing Home Situation in New York State, 1956–78 95

Figure 4.2 Percent of *New York Times* Articles Dealing with Criminal Aspects of the Nursing Home Situation in New York State, 1956–78 96

Figure 4.3 Organizational Chart of the Office of the Special Prosecutor 98

Figure 4.4 The Medicaid Kickback Scheme 103

Figure 4.5 Recoverable Medicaid Funds as of December 31, 1979 107

Figure 4.6 Qualitative Shifts in Patterns of Control of Health Care Providers 124

Figure 5.1 Increase in Number of Nursing Home Beds in New York State, 1966–78 144

List of Tables

Table 2.1   Nursing Home Closings, 1967–74   23
Table 2.2   Investigations of Nursing Home Administrators
            by the Board of Examiners   29
Table 2.3   Guidelines for the Development of a New Code   47

Table 3.1   Cost Ceilings for Facilities, Based on Ratings   79
Table 3.2   Ratings for Skilled Nursing Facilities   82
Table 3.3   Ratings for Skilled Nursing and Health-related
            Facilities   83
Table 3.4   Comparative Costs per diem of Skilled Nursing
            and Health-related Facilities, by Ownership,
            1974   87

Table 4.1   Budgets for the Office of the Special
            Prosecutor   100
Table 4.2   Staffing Levels in the Office of the Special
            Prosecutor at the Beginning of the Calendar
            Year   101
Table 4.3   Cost Disallowances by Reimbursement Category
            for Proprietary Nursing Homes, 1969–75
            Cost Reports   105
Table 4.4   Chronology of Investigations and Reform
            Efforts Related to the New York Nursing
            Home Industry   123

Table 5.1   Status of Patient Abuse Reports Made to
            the Office of Health Systems Management   136

Table 5.2   Action Taken on Completed Investigations of
            Patient Abuse Reports   137
Table 5.3   Completed Investigations of Patient Abuse
            Reports   139

Acknowledgements

It is difficult to acknowledge everyone who helped in the completion of this project because the acknowledgements might be longer than the report. Many people freely gave of their time.

Of particular importance were the respondents themselves, who because they were assured of confidentiality, must remain anonymous. The role of many of them was far greater than that of the usual respondent in a survey. They provided additional documentation, dug up missing facts, and served as patient tutors, consultants, and editors. While not always pleased about what was written, they treated it with good humor and objectivity and were always supportive and encouraging. They are an impressive, committed group of people. None of them fits the stereotype of pinheaded bureaucrat, avaricious operator, bloodthirsty prosecutor, or paranoid busybody. If this investigation has value, it is largely due to their efforts.

Of particular help in the early stages of this project were the Arkell Hall Foundation and the department of preventive medicine and community health at the University of Rochester, which provided me with the time and the encouragement during the 1975–76 academic year to begin to look at issues related to regulation of health facilities.

The project itself was supported by a grant from the National Center for Health Services Research (Grant number 1 RO1 HS 02694-01). The Center's project officer, John Gary Collins, was understanding and supportive of the many complications in the study that delayed its completion.

A special note of appreciation is due those on the staff of the Department of Health Administration at Temple University who imposed some sense of order over the complex task of completing the report. Tony Albano, program coordinator, helped with proofing. Hope Hillman, Audrey Henry, Karen Lessin, and Elaine Ross assisted at various stages in pulling together the tables and in performing the necessary library research. Departmental secretaries Sally Villar and Cindy Jones assisted in the typing of drafts. The final draft was completed by Shelah Burgess, providing able rapid assistance through the bureau of government and business services of the school of business.

Finally, I would like to thank my colleagues, students, and family for their tolerance of my sometimes frantic schedule and preoccupation with the completion of this project.

Preface

Government regulation has produced many curses from health care providers and many exhortations from public officials. It will be defined broadly here to encompass all external efforts to control or influence providers of health services, whether they are appeals to professional pride, pity, pay, or the threat of prison.

Issues related to the regulation of health care providers have heated up since 1975. In spite of the anti-regulatory rhetoric of the Reagan Administration, concerns about fiscal restraint are likely to make that heat even hotter. Public Law 93-641, the National Health Planning and Resources Development Act of 1974, created a new generation of local health planning efforts. The new planning agencies have proven to be more committed to these objectives than most critics believed they would be. The amount of time and energy needed to get the required approvals for federal reimbursement of new capital expenditures has increased, and the outcomes have been at least marginally altered. On another front, the 1972 Social Security amendments produced substantial changes in the certification of institutions for Medicare and Medicaid. Section 244 called for sample validation surveys of hospitals accredited by the Joint Commission for Accreditation of Hospitals (JCAH) for Medicare certification. Sample validation surveys in 1974 and 1975 identified deficiencies substantial enough for 60 percent of those hospitals surveyed to lose their "deemed status" under Medicare and fall under the direct review and control of federally contracted state Medicare inspection teams (Ellis 1977). The JCAH has since responded with far stiffer actions against noncompliant hospitals in the life safety area, raising new questions about the relative costs and benefits imposed on health facilities by such standards (Johnson 1977).

Concern over health care costs has continued to rise along with the costs. A new federal agency, the Health Care Financing Administration, was created in 1977 in order to exert more effective control over federal health care financing by consolidating federal payment, quality, and cost control activities. Legislation to control hospital costs was a top priority of the Carter administration. These efforts, at least initially, were successfully deflected by a voluntary cost containment initiative offered by the industry. Efforts to impose some federal ceilings on health care expenditures, such as were imposed on the New York State Medicaid program, nevertheless, were continued. Pursuing a different course, the Federal Trade Commission (FTC) has been making forays into the health sector through antitrust action. Its occupational licensure program has focused on state laws for licensing health-related professionals and the appropriateness of these laws in restricting entry (U.S. Congress 1979). The FTC also attacked the American Medical Association's sanctions against advertising and price competition among physicians (Schorr 1978).

Simultaneously, the 1977 fraud and abuse amendments to the Social Security Act (P.L. 95-142, Sec. 17) have produced a chain reaction of federal and state efforts to restrain escalating costs and to eliminate fraud and abuse.

Criticism of regulatory activities has come from provider groups, independent think tanks, and the regulators themselves. Scathing and generally well targeted critiques of the cost, inefficiency, and duplication of regulatory efforts have been produced by the American Hospital Association (1977) and a number of state hospital associations (Kinzer 1977, Hospital Association of New York State 1978, Hospital Association of Pennsylvania 1977). Policy groups have advocated eliminating the command and control strategy of regulation and moving toward more market-oriented approaches to supply, demand, and performance (Acton and Newhouse 1972, Ellwood 1974, Havighurst 1980, McClure 1978, Salkever and Brice 1979, Schlenker and Graber 1972).

In 1978 the Government Accounting Office, in response to a request by Congress, began a systematic review of the costs of regulatory efforts in the health sector. Simultaneously, the President manifested his concern by promulgating Executive Order 12004, requiring an analysis of all significant federal regulations. Such an analysis should include an examination of alternative approaches and should essentially be a cost-benefit study (Hellinger 1979). The Office of Health Regulation, a two-year task force within the Health Care Financing Administration, was set up to review regulations related to health care institutions.

The literature on the regulation of health care provides little guidance in these efforts. Although some recent reviews reflect the increasing public concern with the issues, most of the literature deals with immediate practical concerns. Four general observations can be made regarding the majority of this literature:

1) It tends to be diffuse and descriptive, with little effort toward conceptual synthesis.

2) It is largely ahistorical, often failing to recognize the origins of some of the activities being described.

3) Although the importance is hinted at, little attention has been given its internal organizational dynamics of regulation.

4) Proposed solutions reflect more the ideological predispositions and self-interests of the advocates than any balanced evaluation of the existing process. It is, then, hardly surprising that the American Medical Association has supported the move to establish medical directors in nursing home facilities, that some spokesmen for the voluntary nursing home sector have advocated an end to for-profit homes, that advocates of for-profit homes have argued for deregulation and greater use of market mechanisms to control nursing homes, and that lawyers have been the principal advocates for the use of class action suits.

The problem with many of the more analytical economic studies of regulation is that they tend to be fragmented. They focus on the separate aspects of regulation—certificate of need, standards, reimbursement mechanisms, enforcement—rather than on the interdependencies of these aspects. They often overlook the historical and organizational impediments to some of the courses of action they advocate. A case study of some of the interplay between various aspects of regulation might help clarify research and policy issues. In order for such a case study to be useful, the researchers need to overcome their ingrained biases and try not to prejudge the purposes or effectiveness of such activity.

Nursing home regulation would seem to be a particularly useful area for such a case study. Unlike other elements of the health care sector, nursing homes receive the bulk of their income from public sources. As a result, they are more likely targets of regulation and of public criticism than are other components of the health care sector.

Long-term care and its regulation are of great interest in themselves. The increasing proportion of aging persons in the population requires increasing attention to costs, quality, and access issues of long-term care.

New York State is a particularly useful focus for a study of nursing home regulation. It represents by far the largest, costliest public venture in long-term care: 28 percent of all federal Medicaid funds allocated to long-term care flow into New York State. In 1977 the cost of long-term care amounted to $971 million, more than the total Medicaid budget for any other state except California. New York had the highest per diem skilled nursing reimbursement in 1976 ($42.68), almost twice the national average of $24.04.

Consequently, New York has been a major battleground of efforts aimed at gaining federal compliance with standards. Far more financial resources have flowed into the regulatory process in New York than into that of any other state. The overall costs of New York's survey of standards compliance are far higher than those of any other state, although progress toward lowering these costs has been made recently.

New York has long been a trend-setter in health-related programs and in health care regulation. The original Social Security legislation of 1935, which did much to shape the structure of the long-term care sector in the United States, was modeled after earlier New York legislation (Thomas 1969, p. 50). New York was the first state to adopt certificate-of-need legislation and state-controlled prospective rate-setting for both Medicaid and Blue Cross. Its initiatives in regulating the nursing home industry in 1975 set off similar efforts in at least sixteen other states and sparked initiatives to control fraud and abuse at the federal level. New York was also able to avoid bankruptcy through stringent controls on its Medicaid program, in a fiscal crisis far more serious than faced by any other state to date.

In short, nursing homes, particularly the nursing homes in New York State, are on the cutting edge of many changes in regulation within the health sector. A case study of these changes would be worthwhile in considering future regulation of health care in general.

The material synthesized in this report was obtained from a variety of sources over a five-year period. The initial phases were informal, exploratory ones, motivated more by general curiosity than by any desire to complete a specific product. The author was a visiting faculty member in the Department of Preventive Medicine and Community Health at the University of Rochester during the 1975-76 academic year. With the assistance of a group of graduate students, about twenty local nursing home administrators, the regional Health Department staff, and staff in the regional Office of the Special Prosecutor were interviewed. This was during the height of public attention concerning nursing homes within the state and immediately in the aftermath of the reforms initiated by legislation in the summer of 1975. The proposal that served as the basis for this study was completed in the spring of 1976. During 1977 and 1978, the author was involved as an Intergovernmental Personnel Act Fellow with the Office of Policy Planning and Research of the newly created Health Care Financing Administration in Washington. Part of these activities involved talking to a variety of people and collecting information on the problems involved in the regulation of health care facilities in the Medicare program.

The actual formal interviewing for the study was begun by the author and a part-time research assistant beginning in June of 1978. The interviews were open-ended and lasted from forty minutes to over three hours. Before beginning the interviews, respondents were informed of the purpose of the study and were requested to give signed consent. Given the sensitivity of some of the issues, the cooperation was gratifying. In only two cases were we unable to complete interviews.

Our list of respondents was essentially a "snowball sample," with each respondent giving us the names of others whom they felt would be important to contact, given the objectives of the study. We went first to the more visible individuals in the State Health Department, on the staff of the legislature, and nursing home associations. Each person contacted gave us additional names. The list grew, but very often the same names would reappear. A total of eighty persons were formally interviewed. They included representatives of voluntary and proprietary nursing home interests, consumer advocates, legislative staff, and regulators concerned with the various aspects of control described in the chapters of the report. While many more individuals could have been included, the objective of making sure that the different points of view were represented and that those with the appropriate expertise were consulted seemed to be reasonably met.

Rough drafts of sections of the report were completed sometimes in conjunction with follow-up telephone conversations with key respondents. These drafts were then circulated to those who had been most directly involved in the content of the sections. Some responded in writing. Others were followed up either by telephone or in person. The subsequent revisions corrected factual errors and eliminated some of the more subjective or unsubstantiated observations of either the author or of those who were interviewed. Except where it appeared essential to the understanding of a section or impossible to conceal, the names of individuals and specific facilities have been excluded.

A number of problems, all too familiar to those who must work with health care regulations on a day-to-day basis, faced the project. First, nothing would stay still. The regulations, the initiatives, the emphases, the legal precedents, the organizational structures, and the actors themselves continued to change. Follow-ups in some cases were hampered by rapid turnovers. Several respondents had changed jobs three times in the course of the year and a half of interviewing. Second, even if everything had changed at a much slower pace, the areas touched on by the study involved many complex technical issues beyond the scope of such a short overview. Finally, it was difficult at times to disentangle facts from the rhetoric of those attempting to present a strong case for the position or interest they represented.

A variety of other sources, in addition to interviews, however, proved helpful. The study had the benefits of the earlier work of both the New York Moreland Act Commission and the Temporary State Commission on

Living Costs and the Economy, as well as of the Office of the Special Prosecutor, whose efforts were summarized in both annual reports and several special reports (Moreland Act Commission 1975-76; Temporary State Commission 1975). Of particular assistance was a study conducted for the Health Department by the Rensselaer Polytechnic Institute (RPI 1979). Articles in *The New York Times* and *Village Voice* for these years proved useful. The Health Department was particularly helpful in supplying information on the operating characteristics of the system over the period of study, including data on reimbursement rates, number of beds, openings and closings of homes, inspection, auditing, and prosecution results, and the charge and collection of fines.

A study by Bruce Spitz on capital cost reimbursement for nursing homes in New York was also useful (Spitz 1979). William C. Thomas's book on the early history of nursing home regulations in New York was invaluable in putting the present events in perspective (Thomas 1969).

These respondents and materials, imperfect, incomplete, and in a few cases, perhaps, self-serving, formed the basis of this book. It should be read with skepticism and, also, hopefully, with some tolerance for the time and resource constraints imposed in pulling it together.

The book is organized into six chapters. The first provides the history of the regulatory offensive in New York. The next four focus on strategies of control and attempt to assess their effectiveness in New York: professional standards enforcement, rate setting and reimbursement, criminal prosecution, and consumers. Chapter Six summarizes some of the possible lessons of this experience for the health sector as a whole.

Chapter One

Nursing Homes on the Cutting Edge

Emergence of Professional Controls

At the turn of the century, the only real controls over the health sector were the individual consciences of providers and the willingness of the general public to pay for their services or products. Medicine was fragmented into rival factions with conflicting doctrines. State licensing laws were largely ineffective in assuring a minimal level of competence. A hospital could be any building one wished to label as such. There were no standards. Proprietary schools dominated the training of physicians. Most medical schools were open to high school graduates, and many waived even this requirement. Many of the proprietary schools were operated primarily as profit-making businesses. Instruction within them often consisted of nothing more than a series of large lectures, and students graduated without ever hearing the heartbeat or feeling the pulse of a patient. The more marginal schools were diploma mills, which found it lucrative to exploit the aspirations of the disadvantaged. Abuses within the profession itself were rampant. Fee-splitting, or kickbacks, were an accepted way of life. Fortunes were made by charlatans for quack cures.

As the scientific basis of medicine grew, the influence of its practitioners grew as well. Professional controls become possible only when those pressing for them can make a persuasive argument for their social usefulness. That point apparently was reached about 1910 or 1912, when "it became possible to say of the United States that a random patient with a random disease consulting a doctor at random stood a better than fifty-fifty chance of benefiting from the encounter" (Henderson 1961, p. 136). A methodical housecleaning began. Entry into the medical profession was restricted, training standards were raised, hospital conditions were improved, and attempts to police the ethics of medical practice were increased.

In 1901 the American Medical Association (AMA) began to collect data on medical education, and a thirty-year campaign to raise medical school standards began. With the AMA's creation of the Council on Medical Education in 1904, the effort accelerated. Only 82 of the 161 schools surveyed by the Council in 1907 were found acceptable. Although that report was never released, the AMA worked closely with the Carnegie Foundation in encouraging Abraham Flexner's more systematic study of medical education. The Flexner report, published in 1910, largely reflected changes that had already begun. The changes represented a consolidation of control over medicine by allopathic physicians with the support of corporate philanthropy, such as the Rockefeller and Carnegie foundations (Berliner 1975). The support of scientific medicine fit the conservative orientation of these foundations. It focused attention on technological, rather than social or political, solutions to what were essentially social problems. Between 1904 and 1920, the number of medical schools dropped from 160 to 88, and the number of graduates dropped from 5,747 to 3,047 (Rayack, 1967, pp. 69–70). Fifty-one medical schools were closed and fifty-one were merged. The AMA's Council on Medical Education assumed major responsibility for upgrading medical education; it has since exerted a powerful influence on such training and, as a consequence, on the health sector as a whole. The Council approves undergraduate medical schools, internship and residency programs, continuing medical education, and a variety of training programs in allied health professions. Such approval of training is a condition of professional licensure in most states. Since much of such training goes on in settings where care is delivered, the Council also controls the way such services are structured. Critics have argued that the council's initial concerns with improving education have been replaced by more narrow concerns of restricting entry and protecting the financial position and authority of physicians (Freidson 1970, Rayack 1967, Freidman 1962, Kessel 1958).

Perhaps more important to the emergence of professional control of institutional care were the activities of the American College of Surgeons. Established in 1913 as an independent professional association, the College faced the immediate problem of determining who was eligible for membership. It was decided that review of a surgeon's work was an essential condition. The College discovered, however, that few hospitals kept such records, so review proved to be impossible.

Concerned with improving the standards of hospital surgical practices, the American College of Surgeons began a program to survey hospitals. The initial standards for approval, drawn up by a committee chaired by Ernest Codman, included what Codman described as "end result analysis" to determine whether the treatment was as effective as possible (Cristoffel, 1976). In its first survey, in 1918, the College found that of 692 hospitals with more than 100 beds, only 89 met their minimum standards. The findings were so appalling, particularly since many of the leading medical centers in the country had failed the test, that all copies of the report were burned and the initial criteria were scrapped. For both political and practical reasons, end result analysis was not included in subsequent versions of the minimum standards. Emphasis was placed on structure of records, procedures, and paper. Only since the 1970s has there been renewed interest in what Codman advocated (Cristoffel 1976).

In 1920 the College published the first list of hospitals that met the watered down standards. Of the 671 hospitals with more than 100 beds, 392 either met the standards at the time of inspection or, after making up deficiencies in one or more areas, met the standards later. The revised minimum standards included the following items (American College of Surgeons 1920, pp. 642–43):

1. That physicians and surgeons privileged to practice in the hospital be organized as a definite group or staff. Such organization has nothing to do with the question as to whether the hospital is "open" or "closed," nor need it affect the various existing types of staff organization. The word *staff* is here defined as the group of doctors who practice in the hospital inclusive of all groups such as the "regular staff," the "visiting staff," and the "associate staff."

2. That membership upon the staff be restricted to physicians and surgeons who are (a) competent in their respective fields and (b) worthy in character and in matters of professional ethics; that in this latter connection the practice of the division of fees, under any guise whatever, be prohibited.

3. That the staff initiate and, with the approval of the governing board of the hospital, adopt rules, regulations, and policies governing the professional work of the hospital; that these rules, regulations, and policies specifically provide:

   a. That staff meetings be held at least once each month. (In large hospitals the departments may choose to meet separately.)

   b. That the staff review and analyze at regular intervals the clinical experience of the staff in various departments of the hospital, such as medicine, surgery, and obstetrics; the clinical records of patients, free and pay, to be the basis for such review and analyses.

4. That accurate and complete case records be written for all patients and filed in the hospital, a complete case record being one, except in an emergency, which includes the personal history; the physical examination, with clinical, pathological, and X-Ray findings when indicated; the working diagnosis; the treatment, medical and surgical; the medical progress; the condition on discharge with final diagnosis; and, in case of death, the autopsy findings when available.

5. That clinical laboratory facilities be available for the study, diagnoses, and

treatment of patients, these facilities to include at least chemical, bacterio-
logical, serological, histological, radiographic, and fluoroscopic service in
the charge of trained technicians.

The inspection process proceeded cautiously and diplomatically. Having
no legal sanctions, it relied on persuasion and the goodwill of the institutions. The hospital "visitors," as they were called, were carefully instructed
[American College of Surgeons 1920, p. 544 (italics added)]:

> The visitor is to collect facts and he is to collect facts only with the good will
> and approval of the respective hospitals. His mission is business. He is not a
> detective, an unbidden critic, nor a social caller. *He is not to make com-
> parisons of one institution with another.* He is to be helpful and constructive.
> The success of his visit will depend much upon his sincerity. He must *believe* in
> his work. The visitor who is unwelcome has in all probability not wisely
> handled the situation.

Hospitals were notified several months in advance of visits. Widespread
cooperation with the program was reported. As one physician is reported to
have said, "It is wise that we lead now in a program for better care of
patients rather than be forced later by the public to follow such a program"
(American College of Surgeons 1920, p. 544). That argument has echoed
and reechoed in debates over professional control until the present.

As a result of the American College of Surgeons' efforts, procedures for
controlling the basic quality of care in institutions became accepted within
the health sector. In the 1920s the procedures were to become more
elaborate, the standards higher and more precise, but the basic structure
and strategy remained unchanged. It was not inevitable that regulation
would take the form it did: It could have taken on more of the scientific
precision that Codman advocated, or it could have become a public
responsibility rather than that of a private professional organization. The
form that it did take, however, had an extremely important influence on the
development of health care.

The thirty-year campaign by the American College of Surgeons to improve hospital standards produced impressive results. Institutions were
transformed from chaotic, motley, often archaic structures into modern
hospitals. Duties and procedures assumed a degree of predictability across
institutions for various professional staff. Malcolm MacEachern, director
of the College's hospital standardization program, became known as the
father of modern hospital administration, and his book, *Hospital Organization and Management*, first published in 1935, was known as its bible. The
book remained the major text for hospital administration students and the
key reference of practitioners for almost thirty years.

The standards program was one of the driving forces behind changes in the financing of hospital care as well. More complex institutions adapting to more rigorous professional expectations were more costly. They required a more reliable, uninterrupted flow of income than was possible through reliance on charitable contributions and the uncertain ability of patients to pay. Hospitals were undergoing a simultaneous transformation from chari- table institutions designed primarily to serve the indigent, as had been their mission since the Middle Ages, to institutions serving the broader popula- tion. That transformation was accelerated by the American College of Surgeons' efforts to upgrade hospitals. Reflecting the same aversion to public control that had spurred the voluntary standards program, the first efforts of hospitals to achieve a reliable flow of income were local, volun- tary hospital-sponsored insurance plans or local Blue Cross plans, which were established in the 1930s. The inability of these private insurance pro- grams to assure an income that would meet the rising costs of improved standards of care and rapidly developing technology eventually produced the Medicare public insurance program for the elderly in 1965, and it con- tinues to produce pressure for a broader form of national health insurance. The Medicare program's reliance on "fiscal intermediaries," predominantly Blue Cross plans, to reimburse hospitals and physicians reflects the continu- ing desire of providers of health care to insulate themselves from public control.

The College's campaign also focused on physicians. It sought to end fee splitting and to restrict surgical privileges in hospitals. The latter efforts sometimes brought them into conflict with general practitioners and the AMA.

By 1950 the financial burden of the hospital surveys had become too great, from the point of view of the College, to be sustained from the dues of its members. After a good deal of professional association infighting, the surveys were taken over in 1952 by a new body, the Joint Commission on Accreditation of Hospitals (JCAH). The JCAH represented the American College of Surgeons, the American College of Physicians, the American Hospital Association, the American Medical Association, and the Canadian Medical Association. At the time, 3,352 of the 4,111 hospitals with more than twenty-five beds had met the standards for accreditation (Davis 1960, p. 388).

The new accrediting body adopted the methods and procedures of its predecessors. Reflecting the new professional interests represented in the JCAH, both adequacy of institutional administration and the quality of nursing care were now included as criteria for accreditation. Efforts to ex- pand JCAH activities to the accreditation of nursing homes were under- taken, but these efforts have proceeded slowly. At present, only 7 percent

(1,300 out of 18,900) of all United States nursing homes are accredited by the JCAH (Joint Commission of the Accreditation of Hospitals 1979; National Center for Health Statistics 1980). In New York State, 20.7 percent (162 out of 783) of all nursing homes are JCAH-accredited (New York State Department of Health 1980). The bulk of these are either sections of hospitals or are owned by hospitals.

Emergence of Public Regulation

Public regulation has emerged even more slowly than professional controls and is still very much in their shadow. Although the licensing of physicians dates back to the nineteenth century, the licensing of institutions did not really begin until after World War II. At that time fewer than a dozen states had hospital licensure laws, and most of them were toothless (Somers 1969, p. 102).

Public regulation of health institutions originated mainly in the child welfare movement of the mid-nineteenth century. This movement consisted of sporadic efforts to pressure states into controlling the appalling conditions in almshouses and asylums for abandoned children. The first licensure legislation was an amendment to the New York State Constitution in 1894 requiring that private facilities caring for children be certified by a state board of charities in order to be eligible for payments from local governments (Somers 1969, p. 102). The Social Security Act of 1935 gave additional impetus to the child welfare movement: it required those using Title V funds (money for maternal and child health, crippled children, and child welfare activities) to follow standards drawn up by the federal agency created to administer this program, the Children's Bureau. As a result, by 1944 thirty-eight states had laws concerning licensure of maternity sections of hospitals. Maternity regulations have remained strong in many state hospital licensing programs (Somers 1969, p. 103).

The Children's Bureau was the major focus of federal health-related regulatory activities during the late 1930s. Through the 1950s it rivaled the Federal Bureau of Investigation both in political unassailability and discipline.

The Hill-Burton Act of 1946, which provided massive federal matching funds for hospital construction, required states to provide minimum standards of construction, maintenance, and operation for hospitals built with these funds. A 1950 amendment to the Social Security Act required that states must designate a body responsible for "establishing and maintaining standards for such institutions," in order to qualify for federal matching funds in public or private institutions for the care of welfare recipients

(Somers 1969, p. 107). This marked the beginning of the licensing of nursing homes and related facilities. Typically these agencies, generally lodged in the state health department, were charged with the following responsibilities (Somers, 1969, pp. 108–9):

1. Prepare regulations;
2. Review regulations and the basic law from time to time and prepare recommendations;
3. Develop procedures for inspection of facilities covered by the law;
4. Inspect, or cause to be inspected, facilities covered by the law;
5. Issue licenses to facilities found to be in substantial compliance with the law and regulations;
6. When there is found to be substantial non-compliance:
   a. Inform the violator of the minimum requirements which apply,
   b. Supply expert consultative services to assist the violator in identifying the problems involved and the steps necessary to achieve compliance,
   c. Take proper steps to close the facility if no action to comply can be or is taken;
7. Provide educational and consultative services on a regular basis and/or on call: (a) in matters in which licensed institutions have considerable problems in meeting standards; and (b) in those matters not covered by nongovernmental organizations.

In spite of these apparently broad powers, such licensure activity seemed to have little impact on institutions, at least until the mid-1960s. The agencies can be generally characterized as weak, understaffed, and poorly financed. The 1957 edition of MacEachern's *Hospital Organization and Management* does not contain a single mention of these agencies in its 1,300 pages, although, of course, the book devotes a chapter to accreditation. Its 1962 successor, Owen's *Modern Concepts of Hospital Administration*, contains no reference to licensure. Its lengthy chapter on hospital law, although quite thorough and explicit on other issues (for example, the illegality of detaining patients or corpses in order to exact payment of bills), is silent about the legal requirements for licensure (Owen 1962). The 1959 *Hospital Law Manual* does not contain a section on licensure (University of Pittsburgh 1959). One legal expert in the early 1960s who asked several states for a copy of their licensing regulations was told that none of the states could comply because each had only a single copy on file (Somers 1969, p. 109).

It was only with the passage of the Medicare-Medicaid legislation in 1965 that the federal government's laissez-faire attitude toward quality control was explicitly rejected. Until then, almost no requirements for eligibility for federal funds had been imposed on health care institutions*: Any institution was eligible to participate in the public assistance and worker's compensation programs. The Medicare legislation, however, spelled out minimum requirements for eligibility. Echoing the standards established by the American College of Surgeons forty-five years earlier, it specified the maintenance of clinical records, a medical staff with bylaws, twenty-four-hour nursing service under at least a licensed practical nurse, and "such other requirements as the Secretary of Health, Education, and Welfare finds necessary in the interest of the health and safety of individuals who are furnished services in the institution, except that such other requirements may not be higher than the comparable requirements prescribed for the accreditation of hospitals by the Joint Commission on Accreditation of Hospitals" [P.L. 89-97, Section 102(a)]. Hospitals accredited by the JCAH were deemed to have met Medicare standards and required no separate surveys. Because its ability to grant "deemed" status gave the JCAH a quasi-public role, the Social Security Administration attempted to get the JCAH to change its bylaws and appoint public or consumer representatives to its governing board (Bernstein 1977). The JCAH viewed the Social Security Administration's proposal with shock and dismay, and its board rejected the proposal. The Social Security Administration abandoned its efforts to gain public representation on the JCAH.

Utilization review requirements with somewhat different origins were also a part of these standards. Medicaid standards for participation were initially left up to the states and then added to federal requirements in 1970. The JCAH agreed to adopt the utilization review requirements as part of their own minimum standards. In carrying out the intent of Congress, institutional state licensure laws were bypassed as inadequate, and the conditions for participation were based primarily on JCAH requirements. The initial standards were developed after extensive consultation with professional interest groups. The final document was a sixty-four-page manual dealing with conditions of participation. It listed sixteen conditions and outlined a number of standards. Altogether, there were over 100 separate standards and several hundred factors. In most states, HEW contracted with state or local health departments to carry out inspections of hospitals without JCAH accreditation and of nursing homes, which had yet to be included in JCAH accreditation efforts. Such certification functions were

---

*Membership in local Blue Cross plans was made a requirement for some state funds. The Children's Bureau and the Office of Vocational Rehabilitation imposed requirements related to their own programs, but these constraints had little general impact on health care institutions.

generally merged with those sections or bureaus in state health departments that had been responsible previously for institutional licensure.

While public responsibility was assumed, the mission of the Medicare certification program was little different from that of the JCAH or its predecessor, the standardization program of the American College of Surgeons. It was designed as a means of educating and stimulating improvement rather than as a means of exerting strict bureaucratic control. The state health departments and the Social Security Administration encouraged certifying agencies and financial intermediaries such as Blue Cross to assist the institutions in every way possible. Medicare funds were made available for such educational purposes to both the certifying agencies and intermediaries. When Medicare eligibility began on 1 July 1966, the Social Security Administration bent over backward to certify institutions, hoping that later, through persuasion and consultation, it could improve the more marginal institutions (Feder 1977, pp. 10–21). The Public Health Service tried to use the Medicare program as leverage to upgrade facilities by insisting that JCAH standards be the minimum for participation. It lost out to the Social Security Administration's concern with smooth implementation of the Medicare program and access to beneficiaries. The certification process assumed the more tolerant, educational posture of the JCAH, as well as the JCAH's resistance to public disclosure (Feder 1977, p. 25). Ninety-five percent of the applicants and 96 percent of hospital beds had received Title XVIII certification. Only 8 percent of the approximately 2,700 hospitals not accredited by the JCAH were denied such certification (Feder 1977, p. 16). This is hardly an impressive box score, but it is probably more than the number of hospitals that have had their state licenses revoked. The program had relatively little effect on hospitals, since most of them already met JCAH standards. The potential impact of the certification program on nursing homes was far greater. That impact will be assessed in Chapter Two.

While authorities generally lament the ineffectiveness of state regulatory machinery, New York State has been held up as a conspicuous exception (Somers 1969). In 1964 Nelson Rockefeller, concerned with rising Blue Cross rates, set up the Governor's Committee on Hospital Costs, a citizens' group headed by Marion B. Folsom, an executive at Kodak and a former secretary of HEW. The group's major recommendation, that nearly all state functions relating to the regulation of hospitals be transferred to the state Department of Health, was enacted as Article 28 of the Public Health Law in 1965.

As of 1 February 1966, the Department of Health became responsible for supervising and inspecting all hospitals, nursing homes, and related medical facilities.

The Medicaid program, which initially made approximately 45 percent of the state's population eligible, was an intolerable burden to local governments, for, under the New York Medicaid program, they had to pay about 25 percent of its costs. In response to this crisis, reimbursement rates were frozen by legislation in 1969, and a new arrangement was made between providers and the state. This allowed the Commissioner of Health to determine rates based on "efficient production of health services" rather than simply on costs. Such a mechanism was so contrary to the beliefs and conventional wisdom of administrators that they failed to respond effectively and, as a result, had relatively little input into the development of the initial regulations (Elliott 1976). A prospective reimbursement mechanism was established in 1970.

In terms of state regulation of both quality and cost, New York has been one of the most innovative. The regulatory machinery in Article 28 of the Public Health Law provides for the Department of Health, assisted by the Hospital Review and Planning Council, to develop a health facility code and to enforce it. Inspections are conducted by the Office of Health Systems Management interdisciplinary teams, including a physician, an administrator, a nurse, a sanitarian, a social worker, a physical therapist, and a nutritionist. These teams are relatively well paid and, in comparison to other states, many of which may have only a single nonprofessional performing these functions, well staffed.

Emerging Contradictions in Control

Neither the creation of Medicare and Medicaid requirements for participation nor, in New York State, the enactment of Article 28 controls and prospective reimbursement did much to alter the premises upon which controls were based. The JCAH essentially set the standards and, with respect to hospitals, certified them for federal funds. It was also influential in developing nursing home standards. The responsibility for certifying nursing homes, however, was generally absorbed by the state health departments, which were usually eager to get federal funds to subsidize their own licensure efforts. Although conducted by a public agency rather than a professional organization, procedures were almost the same as in the past; controls continued to be predominantly professional in character and in objectives. Public regulations either mirrored professional controls or were little more than paper structures.

Medicare and Medicaid have produced a dramatically different climate. In contrast to the forty years before 1966, during which the public share of total health spending remained fixed at about 25 percent, the public share rose to over 40 percent in the next five years (Cooper and Worthington 1973). However, an elderly individual now pays more uninflated out of pocket for health care than he did before the passage of Medicare. The federal increase in the costs of the Medicare and Medicaid programs absorbs an increasing share of all federal health-related expenditures. The percent of gross national product going for health care has risen from 6.1 percent in 1965 to 9 percent in 1979 (Gibson 1980, p. 12). Projecting some of the more recent rates of increase into the future, one can come to the conclusion that 100 percent of the gross national product will be going for health care before this country's four hundredth birthday. The proportion of health care expenditures going to nursing homes has increased more than 70 percent since 1965 and accounts for almost 8.4 percent of all health care expenditures (Gibson 1980, p. 13). In 1940, expenditures on nursing homes accounted for only .8 percent of all health care expenditures (Gibson 1979, p. 23). There is an impending crisis in the Social Security system as a whole because of shifts in the age structure of the population. As those persons born during the baby boom of World War II approach retirement, they will be supported both in terms of retirement and health benefits by a smaller labor force, one born in years of declining birthrates.

The cost implications of the present trends are most painfully obvious in the nursing home sector of New York State. In 1974, the Medicaid program in New York State paid over 80 percent of nursing home costs. Between 1967 and 1975, Medicaid reimbursement rates for proprietary institutions increased 164.8 percent in contrast to a 132.8 percent rise in per diem rates for hospitals and a 64.3 percent increase in the Consumer Price Index for the New York metropolitan area (Moreland Act Commission 1976 p. 7). In 1975 it cost an average of more than $13,500 per year to maintain a Medicaid patient in a proprietary home; in one voluntary home, the Medicaid cost of such maintenance was over $26,000. Between 1967 and 1975, dramatic changes took place in the care provided in nursing home facilities and in their number and size. As indicated in Figure 1.1, the number of beds in the state increased more than 60 percent between 1965 and 1975.

During that same period, 400 homes, with a total of over 17,500 beds, were closed. Most of these were smaller homes of wood frame construction that did not comply with the fire safety code. Over 44,500 new beds were constructed. The Department of Health's inspection process assisted both in upgrading the quality of care and in escalating the cost of it. Under the prodding of inspection teams, staffs were increased and, at least on paper, nutritionists, physical therapists, and social workers began to play a role in the care of patients. An alliance grew between nursing home operators and their professional staffs and the Health Department's inspection teams, an alliance similar to the one that had often existed between the JCAH and the

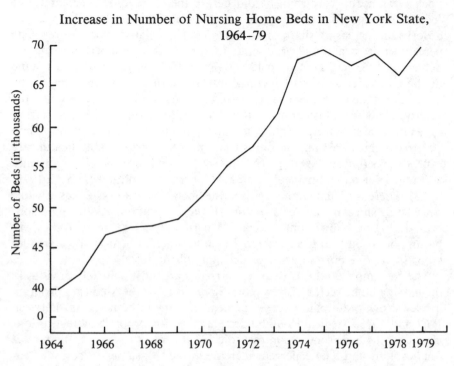

Figure 1.1

Increase in Number of Nursing Home Beds in New York State, 1964–79

Sources: Dunlop 1979; Hynes 1976, 1977, 1978a, 1979; New York State Department of Health 1980.

administrators and professional staffs of hospitals. Some operators proved adept at manipulating this relationship, using the teams as advocates for increased costs and counting on the creation of a professional-collegial atmosphere to produce a reluctance to enforce bureaucratic rules. This relationship contributed to a more than eightfold increase in Medicaid expenditures for long-term care between 1967 ($111 million) and 1975 ($981 million). If one looks at this within the context of the threatened bankruptcy of New York City and the increasingly serious financial problems faced by the state government, it is not hard to understand why questions were asked about what was happening to this money.

The answers to some of those questions produced a regulatory offensive very different from anything that had preceded it. Although this offensive may eventually deal with the entire system, nursing homes are the most vulnerable part of the health sector. They serve a predominantly Medicaid population. They usually lack the political connections provided by influential board members in many voluntary community hospitals. They can not rely on the support of their medical staff in the same way that most hospitals can where the economic interdependency is far greater. Nursing homes are on the cutting edge of changes in control of health care that may well be as significant as those that took place at the turn of the century. It makes sense then to pause, stand back, gain some perspective, and then evaluate the New York State nursing home regulatory experience.

New York State's Regulatory Offensive

The rumblings of battle began to be heard in the spring of 1974. It escalated into a full-scale war conducted at a fever pitch. Few people connected in any way with nursing home affairs in New York State were left unscarred. One operator under investigation committed suicide, half a dozen were sentenced to jail, and many others faced large fines. The reputations of many of the state's political leaders were damaged. The Health Department and its top officials were ridiculed as paper tigers. The proprietary sector of the nursing home industry was portrayed in the early stages as a vulture preying on the old, and its justification for existence was challenged. Later investigations raised questions about the sloppy management and excessive costs of public and voluntary homes. Enough structural changes have taken place to suggest that things will never be quite the same again.

During the summer of 1974, the Temporary State Commission on Living Costs and the Economy began to investigate nursing home real estate transactions, uncovering evidence of what they regarded as massive fraud and windfall profits (Temporary State Commission on Living Costs and the Economy 1975, p. 23). Nursing homes and the financial problems of the elderly had been focuses of the Commission's investigations since its inception in 1973, but from September 1974 until the termination of the Commission in March 1975 these became the sole focus. Public hearings were conducted. Before 1974, the New York State nursing home sector was almost undisturbed by press coverage. Beginning in 1974 and peaking in 1976, as indicated in Figure 1.2, nursing homes were engulfed in a tidal wave of press coverage. Two reporters, John Hess of the *New York Times* and Jack Newfield of the *Village Voice,* produced prolific coverage of the existing problems and abuses of the long-term care system. Both identified widespread fraud and inappropriate influence of political leaders by nursing home interests. Public pressure mounted through the fall of 1974. A flurry of activity followed Governor Hugh Carey's assumption of office in January 1975. His first two acts as governor were the creation of the Moreland

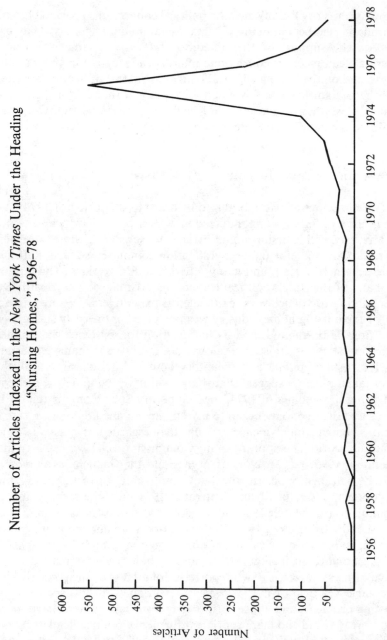

Figure 1.2

Number of Articles Indexed in the *New York Times* Under the Heading
"Nursing Homes," 1956–78

Commission to conduct hearings and make recommendations concerning the nursing home industry and the creation of the Office of the Special Prosecutor to investigate alleged criminal activity and to prosecute, when appropriate. Governor Carey replaced Hollis Ingraham with Robert Whalen as commissioner of the Department of Health. Previously, the job of commissioner had remained detached from the ebb and flow of state politics. Whalen, former deputy assistant health commissioner, was charged with changing the essentially passive, low-profile nature of the department.

The Moreland Act Commission began operations in March with a full-time staff of thirty-six and an annual budget of close to $1 million. The Office of the Special Prosecutor was organized at the same time. It had four regional offices and a budget of approximately $2 million, which was to grow over the next four years to more than $10 million and to encompass a staff of more than 400.

Andrew Stein, chairman of the Temporary State Commission on Living Costs and the Economy, accurately reflected the tone of the early stages of the offensive in a proclamation attached to the front of that commission's final report (Temporary State Commission on Living Costs and the Economy 1975, pp.1–2):

> The dismal picture of venality and inhumanity painted by the proprietary nursing home industry shocked each and every member of the Commission. We found the proprietary nursing home system so riddled with corruption that it may not even be capable of complete reform. Accordingly, even as we strive to introduce desperately needed change, we must simultaneously enlarge and expand our non-profit system of care. It is necessary and proper, even taking into consideration constitutional guarantees, that the proprietary system must end in this state. We cannot and must not continue to place the lives of our infirm elderly under the domination of a proprietary system that has so callously abused its trust.

> We cannot permit ourselves to believe that much publicized investigations will automatically cure the problems of the elderly in nursing homes. Detection is only the first step in the process of reform. The rest of the solution lies in areas of legislative and administrative reform, and tough enforcement of new laws. The Commission has only started the process. It is now up to the public to ensure that their elected officials discharge their responsibilities.

> Now is the time to act. The legislators and the public are aware of the problems of nursing homes. If we now fail to enact effective legislation, we are condemning our infirmed elderly to many more years of suffering to satisfy the greed of private profiteers. Anything less than tough laws from our legislature will amount to nothing more than "politics as usual." I promise to use all of my strength to fight for substantive, not mere cosmetic, change.

Newly appointed Commissioner of Health Robert Whalen announced at the New York State's Proprietary Nursing Homes Association's convention in the Catskills in June 1975 that, from then on, nursing home inspection teams would no longer serve as "consultants" to the homes; they would serve as policemen and regulators. These remarks seemed to characterize the dramatic change in the department that had begun in the fall of 1974. Increasingly, the Health Department and the nursing home operators began to view each other as adversaries.

Placed on the defensive because of charges of influence peddling, the legislature faced intense pressure for stiff legislative action.

Three groups were influential in shaping the legislature's nursing home reform package. An Assembly subcommittee on health care, chaired by Assemblyman Alan Hevesi and appointed by Assembly Speaker Stanley Steingut, began its own series of hearings in April and May. The Temporary State Commission on Living Costs and the Economy disbanded in April, having prepared a set of recommendations. The Moreland Commission, although just beginning operations in 1975, wanted to place its stamp on the pending reform package; it submitted a series of recommendations in the spring. Negotiations between the Moreland staff, Stein, Hevesi's group, and Tarky Lombardi, chairman of the Senate Health Committee, and his staff went on through May, June, and July. The Health Department and nursing home association spokespersons reviewed and commented on various parts of the package but generally played a passive, reactive role in shaping the legislation.

The final nursing home reform bills became law in August 1975. The package included the following provisions *(Laws of the State of New York 1975, pp. 992–1019)*:

1. *Patient Rights Shall Be Protected* — Each nursing home is responsible for distributing and conspicuously posting a written patient bill of rights. New patients and staff will be given a copy. The home is responsible for developing a written plan for staff training to assure the protection of each of these rights.

2. *Inspections Shall Be Unannounced* — There will be at least two inspections of every nursing home each year and at least one of these will be unannounced. Any staff member who discloses the date of any such unannounced inspection shall be subject to a temporary unpaid suspension.

3. *Facilities Shall Be Graded* — The Health Department is required to develop a set of procedures for weighting the importance of various health department standards and for developing a scheme for rating homes in terms of the quality of care provided into not less than five categories. That rating shall be posted conspicuously within the facility.

4. *Rates of Payment Shall Be Related To The Quality of Care* — The Commissioner of Health shall develop regulations that relate the rate of payment for each residential health care facility to the operation and program management of the facility as well as to the quality of the patient care by the facility.

5. *All Controlling Persons Are Liable* — Every controlling person is liable in any personal or class action suit, or to the state for any civil fine, penalty, assessment or damages. A controlling person is anyone who, directly or indirectly, has the ability to direct policies within the home with the exclusion of the Health Department and the Board Members of the facility who have no ownership in the operation.

6. *Ownership Interests Shall Be Fully Disclosed* — A full description of the identity of persons with an interest in the business or property and a full description of transactions between the home and such persons shall be filed annually together with the financial statements of the facility. The reports must be accompanied by a sworn, written statement, attesting to the completeness and accuracy of the information filed.

7. *Survey Reports Shall Be Public* — All facilities will be required to post a summary of the deficiencies noted in the most recent inspection and any action taken by the home to correct these deficiencies in a prominent place within the institution. New applicants to the home are to be supplied, upon their request, with copies of the latest inspection report on the home, as are current residents.

8. *Falsification of Financial Statements Shall Be Punished More Harshly* — All financial information required by law to be submitted to the Health Department must be audited by an independent Certified Public Accountant. The knowing submission of false financial statements known to be false, constitutes a Class E felony. The state may sue for treble damages for fraudulent overstatements of cost.

9. *Graduated Fines For Violations Shall Be Imposed* — The Commissioner of Health was authorized to establish a system of penalties of up to $1,000 per day for continuing violations of rules and regulations pertaining to patient care and up to a 5% reduction in Medicaid reimbursement rates sufficient to collect the penalty.

10. *Operating Certificates May Be Temporarily Suspended* — The Health Department was given the authority to suspend the operating certificate (license) of a home without a hearing for up to thirty days if conditions posed imminent danger to the health or safety of patients. It can prohibit placement of new patients and remove patients, and suspend payment of any government funds.

11. *Class Action Suits Shall Be Encouraged* — A facility that deprives a patient of rights or benefits created for his well-being by federal or state law or pursuant to contract is liable for injuries suffered by the patient as a result

of that deprivation. A minimum for compensatory damages was set at one quarter of the facility's daily Medicaid rate per patient for each day that the patient's injury exists. Punitive damages may also be assessed where the facilities' actions are found to have been willful or in reckless disregard of the lawful rights of the patients. These damages are exempt from determination of Medicaid eligibility and need not be applied toward the payment of medical services. In addition, the court may award attorney fees. Insurance that covers such a liability will not be a reimbursible expense.

12. *Additional Recommendations* — A number of additional legislative recommendations and refinements have been made in 1976 by the Moreland Commission. These included the recommendation that legislators and legislative employees be prohibited from representing nursing home clients before state agencies and requiring them to disclose their interests in activities and entities subject to the jurisdiction of the Department of Health, Mental Hygiene and Board of Social Welfare. [This was the only initial recommendation by the Moreland Commission that failed to pass in the wave of nursing home legislation in 1975.] Other recommendations include provisions directing the Commissioner of Health to explore ways to include consumer input into the evaluation of the quality of care in facilities and for the creation of an "Advocate for the Aging" as a part of the State Office of the Aging to serve as a watchdog for patient rights in nursing homes.

On paper at least, these laws represented a combination of the consumer advocate's and the bureaucratic hard-liner's dream. They represented an attempt to create a regulatory environment very different from that advocated by the early pioneers in the American College of Surgeons and different from anything that exists in any other part of the health sector — at least for the time being.

Chapter Two

Tightening Professional Controls

The bulk of control mechanisms in the health sector are professional in character. That is, they rely ultimately upon the subjective judgments of physicians and others with specialized professional expertise. The responsibility for such controls may rest with: (i) organized professional groups within institutions (for example, medical staff); (ii) external professional associations or consortiums of professional associations (for example, the Joint Commission for Accreditation of Hospitals, Council on Medical Education); (iii) publicly funded, but private, professionally controlled external groups (Professional Standards Review Organizations); (iv) publicly organized, but professionally guided groups that control entry into the field (licensure boards, certificates of need); and (v) public groups responsible for standards of care largely defined by professional groups (the Medicare Standards and Certification Program).

The relationship between subjective professional consensus concerning good and bad standards of practice and the mechanism of control becomes more attenuated as one proceeds down this list. The control process takes on a more bureaucratic tone in terms of paperwork and written regulations. This, however, is more a function of the size of these operations than of their intent. The underlying assumptions are the same. The regulating group is essentially dealing with professional colleagues who share the same values and goals. The approach tends to be collegial, consultative, and educational in character. Standards tend to be worded in generalities (for example, "adequate", "appropriate") rather than rigidly (for example, 2.5 nursing hours per patient or three-hour fire resistant construction). They tend to be worded in "shoulds" rather than "shalls." Collegial courtesy governs the interactions between the regulator and the regulated: unannounced inspections violate such notions of professional courtesy and trust. The reviewer is supposed to act not as a regulator, but as a consultant. Persuasion and education are seen as the most appropriate means for upgrading standards and assuring compliance. These assumptions were challenged in New York by the nursing home exposés of 1974.

New York State has been generally recognized as a leader in the development of standards for nursing homes (Somers 1969, p. 110). In 1965, shortly before the passage of Medicare and Medicaid, New York's Article 28 brought about sweeping changes. The state Health Department became responsible for licensing standards in all health-related facilities within the state. The Health Department was also given the authority to license new facilities on the basis of demonstrated public need, the character and competence of the operators, and the financial viability of the facilities. The state nursing home code that went into effect in June 1966 borrowed heavily from the New York City code. This was one of the only changes implemented as a result of the 1958 investigations of proprietary homes by the City's Department of Investigations. The Health Department utilized the New York City code, reviewed other state and municipal codes, as well as the Hill-Burton regulations, and consulted with state medical associations and nursing home associations. The Health Department task force that was established to pull all of these diverse materials together had on it representatives of the medical, nursing, social work, and engineering divisions within the Department. It was assisted by the efforts of a previous interagency task force, put together by the Department of Social Services, to achieve greater uniformity among standards for nursing home care.

The code went into effect in June 1966, shortly before the Medicare program became operational. Survey teams from the old Board of Social Welfare, now under the direction of the Health Department, began to inspect facilities shortly thereafter. Inspections in New York City and some counties continued to use local health department inspection teams under contract to the state; this practice was gradually phased out. The focus of control, the standards, and the dollars to support the effort had shifted, however, from the municipalities to the state. Federal Medicare and Medicaid standards required that facilities meet all state and local licensure requirements. Thus, in theory, at least compliance with the code was incorporated into the certification process.

The organization of the enforcement activities was as ambitious as the code itself. Unlike most states, which initially used generalist surveyors, some of whom had only high school educations, New York adopted a multidisciplinary team approach. The team consisted of a physician, nurse, sanitarian, social worker, administrator, and dietician. Federal funding helped to support these efforts. Indeed, federal contract responsibilities have accounted for the bulk of activities undertaken by the Health Department in surveying facilities. All costs of surveying skilled nursing facilities for the

Medicare program were reimbursed by the federal government. A time and effort reporting system to the regional offices of HEW provided for full payment of the activities of the Office of Health System Management survey teams related to this effort. Since 1972 all of the direct costs of the Medicaid survey were borne by the federal government.* In this case, funds came to the Department of Social Services, which was designated the single state agency responsible for the administration of the Medicaid program. The certification activities were subcontracted to the Health Department, and the costs of this subcontract were submitted along with Department of Social Services quarterly requests for federal Medicaid funds.

While New York State's survey costs are substantially higher than those of any other state, HEW has only recently begun to examine them. The annual Medicaid inspection bill, which reached $9.25 million in 1977, was buried in the multi-billion dollar cost of the New York State Medicaid program (Respondent 1 1978). Thirty-six million dollars in federal Medicaid and Medicare contract payments to the state Health Department between 1971 and 1976 were audited, and about $4.5 million were identified as having been inappropriately spent (Respondent 1 1978). Much of this spending was related to the certification activities of the Health Department. In effect, until the last couple of years, the Health Department inspection process operated on a cost-plus basis similar to that of the industry as a whole. During this period, inspectors served as consultants to the homes. Indeed one respondent mentioned his use of them in constructing a facility. The surveyor also assisted homes in getting altered reimbursement to accommodate the changes they recommended. Recommendations for rate increases to accommodate improvements were routinely accepted by the Bureau of Health Economics (Respondent 47 1978). The relationship of surveyors with their professional counterparts in the facilities were friendly and cordial. If not idyllic, this period was one of relatively high surveyor morale; new institutions were being built, and concrete changes were taking place as a result of their recommendations. It is a period remembered with nostalgia by the surveyors who were interviewed.

Problems with enforcement of standards began to surface with the initiation of more aggressive enforcement activities in 1971. New York, having the highest annual Medicaid expenditure for nursing home care, became a

---

* The federal government fully reimburses each state for those Medicaid activities directly attributable for the survey and certification of skilled nursing and other long-term care facilities. Excluded are costs related to state licensure programs, indirect costs, and other costs, such as equipment and supplies. Indirect costs, equipment, and supplies are reimbursed at 50 percent, the overall reimbursement rate for Medicaid administration in most states (Respondent 1 1978).

focus of federal enforcement efforts. These efforts focused on obtaining compliance with the NFPA Life Safety Code. The New York State Department of Health, concerned with creating a precedent that could be used by noncomplying homes as a defense against future actions, notified 150 noncomplying nursing homes that they would have to correct their deficiencies within six months or their Medicaid provider agreements would be terminated. A class action suit by the affected homes, the Maxwell Case, resulted in a court ruling that each individual case must be reviewed on its own merits and that appropriate appeal procedures would be provided to each home (*Maxwell* v. *Wyman* 1972).

These reviews involved administrative hearings within the Health Department with a department-appointed hearing officer; if unsatisfied, the nursing home could still appeal through an Article 78 procedure, whereby an individual may appeal a ruling by a state administrative agency in the state courts.

In 1972, due to federal pressure, the state Health Department assumed responsibility for physical plant inspections of New York City proprietary nursing homes, after which an additional twenty-eight facilities were given similar six-month notices to correct deficiencies. The Office of Nursing Home Affairs, created in late 1971 to implement the nursing home enforcement initiatives of the Nixon Administration, served as the impetus for these new state activities. Another class action suit, the Hayden Manor case, was begun. However, the passage of P.L. 92-603 (amendments to the Social Security Act) in October 1972 again changed the rules of the game. Authority to waive the Life Safety Code requirements was transferred from the state to the secretary of HEW. Yet, following the Maxwell precedent, the state Health Department was ordered to hold hearings prior to termination of provider agreements. The state was directed by HEW to terminate provider agreements for several other homes. The homes brought action against the Commissioner of Social Services for contempt and finally, in March 1975, the motion to punish for contempt was denied. Decertification proceedings are now, more than twelve years after the life safety requirement was enacted, almost complete. Most of the 150 homes listed in the initial 1971 notification have been closed.

In 1973, a new wave of enforcement activities was begun as a result of an amendment to Article 28 that transferred all responsibility for monitoring standards in New York City proprietary homes to the state Health Department.

The Department was ill-prepared for all of these adversary proceedings and fared poorly in a number of the initial hearings. Its staff resources were strained, and it was reluctant to get involved in combating homes on the imprecise standards of quality of care. Initially, only two attorneys were assigned to such enforcement activities within the Health Department. In those pressured times, the department often attempted to act on incomplete and sometimes inaccurate information. A respondent recalled that in one of the first life safety hearings the Health Department's attorney was placed in the position of trying to prove that a cinder block facility was a wood frame dwelling. As a result, lawyers for operators, convinced that the Health Department didn't know what it was doing, became extremely litigious (Respondent 18 1978). As indicated in Table 2.1, most of the homes that

Table 2.1

Nursing Home Closings, 1967–74.

Bed size	Proprietary	Voluntary	Public	Total
≤50	251	31	9	291(85.8%)
>50≤100	18	9	9	36(10.6%)
>100	4	4	2	12 (3.6%)
Total	273(80.5%)	44(13%)	22(6.5%)	339(100%)

Source: New York State Department of Health Office of Health Systems Management, personal communication, 1979.

were closed were small "Ma and Pa" proprietary operations, many serving the more rural areas. There was little public support and bad local press concerning the Health Department's efforts to throw out "the little guy" who provided a small, caring, home-like environment, as illustrated by the following letter to the editor of a local paper (Cooros 1971):

What are you doing New Year's Eve? Would you and all the residents of Monroe County like to cancel your previous plans and join the 10 non-conforming nursing homes in Monroe County? There won't be any liquor, balloons or an orchestra but there will be dancing. The dancer will be the geriatric patient, who is literally being pushed out on the street by New York State.

You see, we aren't built right. We aren't fire-resistant — but check out with the fire departments as to how often they have answered a fire-call for one of us. Our hallways aren't eight feet wide but more love and compassion travel down our narrow pathways than any 8–10 foot one. Ours expand with all the tender loving care one could desire and need, not by a carpenter's tool!

New York State requires that any new nursing home have at least 60 beds. They don't want us smaller nursing homes around anymore. This is a cruel decision made by political bigwigs in Albany. Don't they realize that these patients primarily exist on large dosages of TLC (nurses' terminology for tender love care)? All the advancement of medical research cannot and never will replace TLC! I will debate anyone who doubts me.

This the small nursing home can do. We can give a personal touch to everyone who enters the home whether it be a doctor right on down to the grocery man. (The patients feel it most.)

Mr. Rockefeller will let a gasoline station or apartment house be built on every vacant lot that's available so long as it is on a competitive basis. But not a nursing home. Oh no, one has to go through years of red tape before one gets this privilege. Why? I wish someone could answer.

See you at our ball on New Year's Eve. Attending will be approximately 300 guests. They won't be looking for a partner to dance with, only a place to live.

I hope when the day arrives that the political and so-called health officers (the ones who are making and enforcing our strict State Hospital Code) need a bed in a nursing home, that they are cared for as individuals and not numbers. This is what happens when everything is allowed to expand to such a large dimension.

The Health Department was not equipped by staff or inclination to throw itself wholeheartedly into adversary proceedings against the homes. The desire for a low-profile professional consultative relationship to the industry was strong. Such a relationship works if those involved share the same values and value the high opinions of their professional colleagues. Such was not always the case.

During the fall of 1974 and into 1975, articles in the *Village Voice* and *The New York Times* and hearings by the Temporary State Commission on the Living Costs and the Economy documented abuses of patients similar to the horrors that had preceded them. Cases of unsanitary conditions, unsafe facilities, the physical assault on patients by staff, and bedsores the size of grapefruits were presented. Both the Temporary and Moreland commissions documented the inability of the Health Department inspection process to control such abuses (Moreland Act Commission 1975, Temporary State Commission on Living Costs and the Economy 1975). Few measurable consequences of uncorrected deficiencies could be documented. The Temporary Commission pointed to political collusion, through which bureaucrats discouraged aggressive stances by surveyors. The Moreland Commission referred to the inspection program as the "Paper Tiger," and challenged both the underlying assumptions that guided the development of standards and the process of enforcement.

Regulatory Changes

Legislative Initiatives

The nursing home reform legislation of 1975, the combined product of the Assembly and Senate health committees and the Temporary and the Moreland commission recommendations, produced four key changes in professional controls:

1. Character and competence of operators (Chapter 656) — The character and competence of operators or any parties with a controlling interest in the operations of a proposed facility must be detailed for the previous ten years and must have maintained a consistently high level of care in order to obtain approval from the public health council for certification.

2. Unannounced inspections (Chapter 653) — Nursing homes must be inspected by the New York State Health Department at least twice yearly. At least one of these inspections must be unannounced. Any employee who gives unauthorized advance notice of an inspection will be penalized.

3. Graduated fines (Chapter 660) — A system of penalties of up to one thousand dollars per day for continuing violations of rules and regulations pertaining to patient care shall be developed with the facility having thirty days to correct the deficiency before a penalty would be assessed.

4. Suspension or limitation of operation certificate (Chapter 657) — The operating certificate of a facility may be suspended for a period of up to thirty days when the Department finds a condition which poses imminent danger to the health and safety of any patient. The facility could be prohibited from or limited in accepting new patients and present patients could be removed. Provision is made for reinspection and withdrawal of suspension or limitation after deficiencies are corrected.

Administrative Initiatives

The stance of the Health Department changed dramatically in 1975. Inspectors were instructed by the newly appointed commissioner, "You are no longer consultants, you are now policemen." Directives to the regional offices requested that homes with serious operational deficiencies be identified. Legal staff was added to deal with enforcement, the organizational structure was modified to deal with some of the problems of coordinating activities and control, and a task force was established within the department to review and develop a code that would move away from nit-picking paperwork and towards an emphasis on outcomes and performance, as recommended by the Moreland Commission. The character and competence review for prospective operators began to be implemented at the same time as the Board of Examiners of Nursing Home Administrators began to act on information obtained from the Office of the Special Prosecutor, Health Department inspectors, and the press.

Results

Restricting Entry

The 1975 character and competence legislation required that any individual listed in an application for an operating license of any facility be reviewed. That review was to take into account the last ten years of experience in the field, and each individual was to demonstrate that he or she had been associated with a "consistently high level of care." The review requirements proved to be exceedingly time-consuming, cumbersome, and of doubtful effectiveness, according to most respondents in the Health Department.

The approach required that regional office reviews by surveyors be forwarded to the central office. Initially, there was no additional staff to perform these activities.

The process affected all facilities, not distinguishing between voluntary and proprietary facilities or between hospitals and long-term care facilities in terms of character and competence reviews. The relationship of board members to the voluntary institution is quite different from that of owners to the proprietary home. Any time there was a change in the composition of a board, a review was required. This resulted in an excessive amount of procedural paper-processing with little pay-off in terms of control.

Finally, the standard penalized those with prior involvement in nursing homes. Although the requirement for having provided a "consistently high level of care" was vague, it was intended to expose owners and operators with direct patient care deficiencies. Yet no owner or operator of facilities could escape at least a few "paper" deficiencies in the preceding ten years. Only those with no prior experience could be assured of passing this requirement.

In 1978 a team of three investigators was hired by the Health Department counsel's office, ostensibly to assist in making the reviews more than a ritual. The operation of the investigators is instructive in terms of the contrast between their operations and those of the surveyors.

The investigative team spends most of the time on the road. They visit a facility at odd hours, usually at night. They are armed with cameras and note pads. After meeting with the administrator in charge and politely but firmly refusing an offer of coffee and a Danish, they blitz through the facility in about twenty minutes. They photograph anything that does not appear to be in compliance with the State Nursing Home code and then retrace their steps making careful notes of each possible deficiency they have identified. Their concern is with recall for the witness stand, and not with completing the blanks. They review the list of discharged patients and contact the next of kin of the deceased. In five of the seven initial reviews, they have turned up glaring deficiencies in facilities that received "good — state" ratings from the regional surveyors. As a result, there has been a good deal of hostility and competition between the two groups. The surveyors feel that the investigators are not competent to review the care in the facilities because they do not have the appropriate professional background (Respondent 27 1978):

> The first facility we went in, we came back and we were . . . , well, as I said, we were not prepared for the conditions that we found in that facility . . . it was filthy. When we came out of that facility at the end of the first night, we could hardly talk, our throats were so sore from the odor of urine. Our eyes were watering. We couldn't stop on the way back to the motel for dinner because we smelled so bad. It had permeated our clothes.
>
> We had determined that (I don't remember the exact figure, but I think in a one-year period) the patients in that facility had suffered over 1,000 accidents. When we went in there the first time and came back with these reports, the reaction we got from the Department was, "Well, what the hell do you know? You are a lay person and we have survey teams in these facilities all the time, the rating certificate on the wall says 'good — state' rating and you guys must be a bunch of weirdos."

They have, however, proven to be exceedingly effective witnesses. In contrast, the surveyors, relatively unprepared for cross-examination by high-powered attorneys, often fail to recall, become flustered, and are sometimes driven to tears by a barrage of detailed questions.

The history of efforts at controlling entry through the certificate of need process reveals that the Health Department has been far more effective in controlling the proliferation of nursing home beds than it has been in controlling hospital beds. Need projections are based on empirical ratios developed from surveys in the Rochester and Western New York regions of actual need rather than existing utilization. Most of the hospital beds in New York State existed before the certificate of need legislation was passed in 1964. As a consequence, while growth in the number of nursing home beds has been effectively restrained, the state still has more acute care beds than it needs. Thus, prospective nursing home patients tend to be backed up in hospitals (Respondent 69 1979). The resulting pressure for nursing home beds makes threats of closure for substandard conditions less credible and puts serious limits on the amount of financial pressure the state can place on these institutions.

Control of those who obtained licenses and operated as licensed nursing home administrators did not become a focus of criticism as a result of the investigation in 1974 and 1975. Not having any investigatory staff of its own, the licensing board was dependent on information forwarded to it from other agencies or from the public as a whole. Since very little had been forwarded to it prior to 1974, it had little opportunity to demonstrate its effectiveness or lack thereof.

The origins of nursing home administrator licensure are in striking contrast to those of other health-related professions. Licensing was not the result of any active lobbying by the occupational group itself. Indeed, there was substantial resistance. Testimony before the Senate Committee on Aging in 1965 raised serious questions about the preparation of individuals to be nursing home administrators. A survey of administrators in Massachusetts revealed that only 18 percent had completed college, 20 percent were high school dropouts, and 10 percent had no formal education at all (U.S., Congress, Senate, Committee on Finance 1967, p. 912). The 1967 Social Security amendments mandated a state licensure program for nursing home administrators (P.L. 90-248, Sec. 236). A National Advisory Council on Nursing Home Administrators provided model legislation to implement the intent of this section of the law, but states were given a good deal of flexibility in developing such a program.

In New York State, Article 28D of the Public Health Law spelled out the requirements for the New York program, which went into operation on 1 July 1970.* All administrators were required to be licensed by the Board of Examiners of Nursing Home Administrators. Originally the board consisted of eleven members: three from the voluntary nursing home sector, three from the proprietary, one physician, one nurse, one educator, one hospital administrator, and one consumer or public representative. Subsequent federal regulations prohibited a majority of board members from any one profession, and the number of consumer representatives was expanded to three. Initially applicants were required to have a high school diploma, good moral character, and 100-clock-hour course in nursing home administration in order to qualify for an examination. National norms are used to pass applicants on a multiple-choice test provided by a commercial testing service. Failure rates have ranged from 25 to 46 percent. In addition,

---

*(*New York [Public Health] Law.* Article 28-D, Title 2, sec. 2896.)

100 hours of continuing education are required for relicensure every two years.

The board is required to investigate any complaint made against nursing home administrators. Complaints have come from health department staff, consumers, and the Office of the Special Prosecutor; some situations have come to the attention of the board through the press. Evidence is collected and the board then determines whether a hearing is warranted. If the board votes for a hearing, a Health Department hearing officer is appointed. The respondent, as in other types of administrative hearings, is entitled to counsel, and a transcript is made of the hearing. The hearing officer then makes a recommendation to the board, which, after reviewing the transcript, can accept or reject the hearing officer's recommendation. The total number of investigations undertaken by the board and resulting in disciplinary actions are presented in Table 2.2 and Figure 2.1. Investigations and disciplinary actions resulting in the loss of licenses increased from 1975 to 1978. Less harsh disciplinary actions, limited suspensions, and censures have continued to be the less frequently used sanctions. At the end of 1978, there were 2,884 licenses in New York State still in place. Only approximately one-half of these are registered nursing home administrators. Forty-one lost

Table 2.2

Investigations of Nursing Home Administrators
by the Board of Examiners.

Year	Number of Investigations		Resulting Action
1971–1974	10	3	Negative
		7	Proceedings instituted
		3	Censures
		1	Revocation of license
		1	Forfeiture of license
		1	Surrender of license
		1	Permanent injunction against unlicensed practitioner
1975	39	19	Continuing investigations
		11	Negative
		9	Proceedings instituted
		2	Revocations of license
		1	Forfeiture of license
		1	Surrender of license
		5	In process

Table 2.2 — Continued

Year	Number of Investigations	Resulting Action	
1976	121	31	Continuing investigations
		51	Negative
		39	Proceedings instituted
		3	Referred to Office of Special Prosecutor for criminal action
		1	Censure
		6	Surrenders of license
		5	Forfeitures of license
		24	In process
1977	110	37	Continuing investigations
		36	Negative
		37	Proceedings instituted
		4	Revocations
		2	Forfeitures of license
		2	Surrenders of license
		1	No penalty
		1	Dismissal
		2	Censures
		1	Limited suspension of license
		24	In process
1978	77	28	Continuing investigations
		3	Negative
		46	Proceedings instituted
		12	Forfeitures
		3	Revocations
		1	Suspension
		1	Surrender
		1	Censure
		1	Referred to Office of Special Prosecutor for criminal action
		1	Cease and desist order
		26	In process

Source: New York Department of Health, Board of Examiners of nursing home administrators 1971–78.

their licenses during this period, a revocation rate of approximately 2.8 percent over the last four years. Comparable figures for physicians across the country, based on state reports to the Federation of State Medical Boards over the past four years, appear to be .00027 percent. This figure is probably an underestimate, since some states failed to report. As indicated in Figure 2.2, a jump in revocation of physicians' licenses nationally took

Figure 2.1

Disciplinary Action Taken Against Nursing Home
Administrators by the New York State Board of Examiners

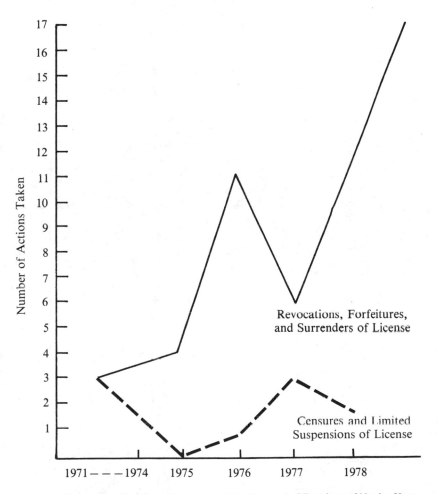

Source: New York State Department of Health, Board of Examiners of Nursing Home
Administration, 1971–78.

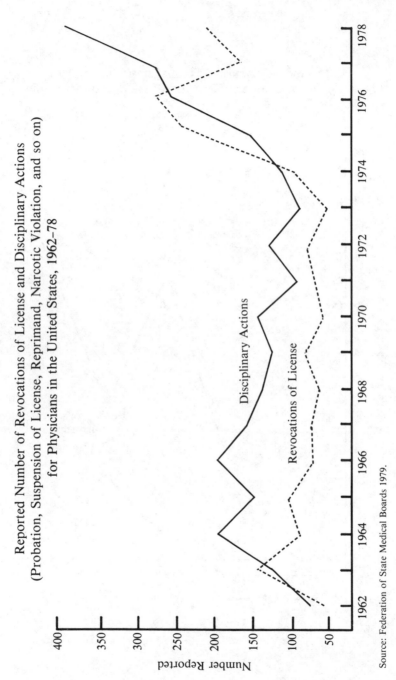

Figure 2.2

Reported Number of Revocations of License and Disciplinary Actions
(Probation, Suspension of License, Reprimand, Narcotic Violation, and so on)
for Physicians in the United States, 1962–78

Source: Federation of State Medical Boards 1979.

place in 1975–76. This jump, however, appears to be primarily the result of improved reporting rather than any increase in disciplinary actions (Respondent 78 1979).

The composition of the board and the continuing education requirements for licensure are almost unique features, although some other professional licensure boards seem to be moving in that direction.

The professional disciplinary process is of limited and only indirect usefulness in controlling standards of care. It is entirely passive. The Board of Examiners of Nursing Home Administrators has no investigative staff and no independent mechanisms for collecting information. The bulk of the disciplinary actions were a result of investigative efforts and prosecution by the Office of the Special Prosecutor. The board's function is to responsibly review complaints against licensed professionals.

Enforcing Standards

All inspections, at least officially, continue to be unannounced. At the same time, regular inspections are rarely a surprise to a facility. Federal Medicare and Medicaid regulations specify a timetable of about three months to allow (i) the facility to respond to the annual certification inspection, (ii) the plan of correction to be reviewed and approved, and (iii) reinspection to assure that the plan of correction has been implemented. Thus, if one takes the date of the agreement and adds nine months, one comes reasonably close to predicting the date of inspection. Periodic Medical Reviews follow a similar pattern. Staffing constraints limit the number of nonroutine inspections that can be done. The emphasis on paper documentation remains. This is not, perhaps, the most efficient way to utilize one's time during surprise visits. The 1975 legislation also requires at least two annual inspections of all homes, regardless of the conditions in the homes or their past record in terms of compliance. Some facilities require many, some none. If a police force patrolled each and every block of a city with the same frequency, regardless of the crime rate, questions would be asked. Efforts to create more flexibility in inspections are being discussed with HEW officials and the state legislature. One concludes that simply making inspections unannounced without increasing their flexibility in terms of frequency and content is ineffective.

In 1975 the Public Health Council aproved a list of fines for 1,053 deficiencies. The fines ranged from one hundred to one thousand dollars a day. One-hundred-dollar fines were levied for such offenses as the failure to include certain information in a service agreement between the nursing home and the patient or his next of kin or sponsor, and unacceptable sampling methods for utilization review. One-thousand-dollar fines included such items as the failure to report institution-related infections immediately to the appropriate health officer, and the failure of the administrator to arrange for opportunities for religious worship and counseling for any patient requesting such services. In theory, an operator who was fined for every possible deficiency on the list would be paying $214,550 daily.

The number of thirty-day fine letters that were written varied by regional office. There was confusion about exactly when such thirty-day fine letters would be appropriate. There was an initial flurry, but then activity of this kind died down.

There was apparently some reluctance on the part of surveyors to utilize such letters of warning or fines. Recommendations for such letters required review by the inspection supervisor, the nursing home review officer, and the area administrator. If the operator failed to comply, there would be an administrative hearing in which the surveyor would be required to testify and would be cross-examined by the operator's attorney.

By the end of 1979, only nine cases had been completed by the Health Department for thirty-day fines. Several things may account for the relatively few hearings that have taken place. First, if a facility has, for example, ten deficiencies, with an average fine of $400 each per day, it would be risking $4,000 if it chose to contest. "No one in his right mind would contest in such a situation" (Respondent 18 1978). Another factor seems to have been the somewhat inconsistent reliance on this tool by the regional health departments. Although instructions concerning which fines were sufficiently significant to warrant thirty-day letters were given, implementation of this policy varied between the regions. In Buffalo, for example, the letters were sent out frequently, while in several other regions relatively little use was made of the letters. They have increasingly fallen into disuse, in part because of several adverse court rulings and in part because of lack of confidence in their efficacy by the area offices. The cost of such hearings is close to $1,000 per day. This led one hearing officer to direct the Health Department and the operators and their attorneys to iron out their relatively minor differences without subjecting all parties to further costly and time-consuming procedures of formal hearings (Respondent 44 1978). So far, the process has produced only $1,000 in actual payment of fines. [Other fines, so-called one-shot fines, which the Health Department presumably had the authority to impose before 1975, have been collected, including a $19,500-fine from one facility (New York State Department of Health).] (Personal Communication, Counsel's Office, 1980)

Some of the hearings were mired down in procedural details. The longest one involved over 3,000 pages of testimony and thirty-four days of hearings, beginning in January 1976 and ending in December 1977. The nursing home operator had not called half of his witnesses and would have preferred to extend the hearing even further. The charges were relatively minor, according to those interviewed. The Commissioner of Health, as of July 1980, had yet to make a final determination, which probably suggests that the recommendations of the hearing officer were not particularly supportive of the Health Department. The Health Department's cost for the hearing was close to $50,000; the operator incurred approximately $100,000 in legal expenses, for which he plans to sue the Health Department when the final determination is made (Respondent 79 1979). The battle continues in spite of the weariness of both sides. At this point, if the fines for the 104 deficiencies identified initially in the inspection report were enforced, they would exceed the yearly income received by the facility. That outcome is unlikely.

Several adverse court decisions have added to the Health Department's frustrations. The entire enforcement effort appears to have lost ground as a result of the creation of the daily fine authority.

In March 1976 the Palatine Nursing Home was charged with 114 violations of the State Hospital Code. Administrative hearings resulted in a determination that Palatine had in fact committed 54 violations, and a total fine of $25,000 was levied. This was appealed through an Article 78 proceeding in the courts on the grounds that the violated regulations are invalid due to their vagueness and subjectivity. An earlier decision, *Levine* vs. *Whalen* (1976, APPDIV) of the Court of Appeals, had struck down other regulations modified by such words as "acceptable," "approved," "permitted," or "determined," since these standards were ruled unreasonable and arbitrary. The Palatine decision, in July 1978, struck down similarly phrased regulations, including "meets the approval or satisfaction of the Commissioner," and "acceptable to the Department." Another provision, stating that construction and equipment standards could be waived by the commissioner if the waiver was in "the community interest," was ruled too vague. It was the court's opinion that such regulations inappropriately gave the commissioner unrestrained discretion regarding those deficiencies. The court decision brings into question the ability to legally enforce much of the existing code.

Since a set of professional standards ultimately rests on the subjective judgment of professionals, the Palatine decision calls into question the ability of any professional standards (such as those of the JCAH, the Council on Medical Education, Medicare, Medicaid) to withstand legal attack. All contain at least some subjective language allowing for professional judgment or discretion. If one succeeds in eliminating such subjectivity, one has also succeeded in completing the evolution from professional to purely bureaucratic standards. In so doing, the rationale of professional autonomy would be destroyed.

The Appellate Division reversed the decision of the lower court in January 1977 concerning the case of a facility that had been fined for deficiencies without being provided a thirty-day period to correct them. The Appellate Division ruled that the more detailed provisions of the 1975 laws superseded the general authority of the Health Department to levy fines, and therefore no fines could be imposed without providing a facility thirty days to correct such a deficiency. While this was clearly not the intent of the legislation, this is the way it was interpreted by the courts. The decision clearly weakened the effectiveness of fines in enforcing standards. Unsanitary conditions, clearly inadequate staff, and conditions that obviously jeopardize the welfare of the nursing home patient can easily be corrected by an operator within thirty days. Clearly these conditions should not have existed in the first place, yet, according to this decision they are not subject to fines. Stated in the most extreme terms, operators can break the law without penalty as long as they don't keep doing it after they are caught. This absurdity was corrected in the 1980 Legislative session by adding clarifying language to the Public Health Law.

The process of adapting to this kind of adversary environment has already begun. Normative professional standards are being translated into bureaucratic ones. For example, standards now specify nursing hours and procedures in more concrete detail than was previously required. It is ironic that such pressures are pushing standards away from what most operators would prefer. The result will be more documentation, more rigidity, and less discretion.

Since the establishment of Article 28 in 1965, the Health Department has had the authority to close a facility that failed to meet its standards. Its experience with the Life Safety Code in the early 1970s demonstrated that such closure could be an exceedingly long, drawn out process. The 1975 law attempted to deal with this in two ways. First, it gave the commissioner the authority to limit or suspend the operating certificate of a facility for up to thirty days without a hearing if there were any "condition or practice or a continuing pattern of conditions or practices which poses imminent danger to the health or safety of any patient." (New York [Public Health] Law, Article 28, Sec. 2806) Second, it set conditions for the replacement of an operator with a receiver. (New York [Public Health] Law, Article 28 Sec. 2801.2) This can be done by the department at the request of the operator, or it can be done by the New York State Supreme Court after an operating certificate has been revoked and the operator has exhausted appeals available to him.

The emergency revocations gained only very limited use. The major problem has been what to do with the patients. Most nursing homes operate at close to full capacity and have waiting lists. The certificate of need controls have been effective — there are no excess beds. In cases where there has been clear and imminent danger, the best the Health Department has been able to do is transfer patients with serious health problems to hospitals, restrict further admissions, and monitor conditions within the facility on a day-to-day basis.

Efforts to remove patients from unsafe, substandard facilities ran into an unexpected roadblock — the patients themselves. Class action suits have blocked the transfer of patients without their consent, without a hearing, and without adequate preparation. Patients and their families have not always sided with the Health Department in its decisions to close facilities.

Facilities continue to be closed, either voluntarily, under pressure from the department, or after the appeal process has been exhausted. All have been primarily for deficiencies in the Life Safety Code. Figures 2.3–2.6 summarize the changes. The closings, described earlier, came in three waves, peaking in 1968, 1972, and 1975. Since facilities opening tended to be substantially larger, there was a net gain in beds in each year. The proportion of proprietary facilities closing has declined relatively little since

Figure 2.3

Openings and Closings of Skilled Nursing Facilities in
New York State by Number of Facilities, 1966–78

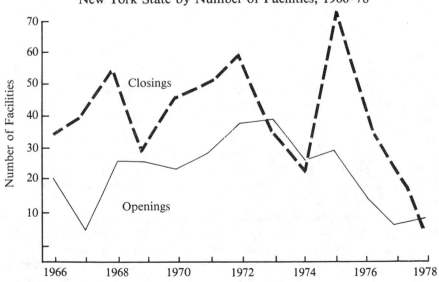

Source: New York State Department of Health 1979.

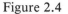

Figure 2.4

Openings and Closings of Skilled Nursing Facilities in
New York State by Number of Beds Gained or Lost, 1966–78

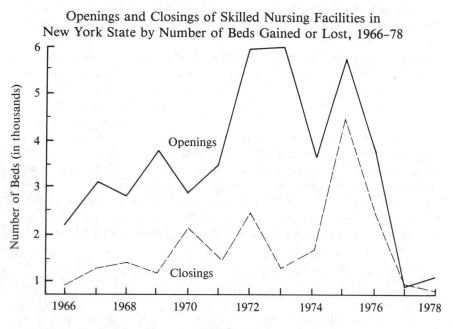

Source: New York State Department of Health 1979.

1966; the proprotion of proprietary facilities opening has declined more
dramatically.

According to the Health Department count in 1979, twenty facilities were
operating with receivers. Six of the facilities were operating under court-
appointed receivers as a result of bankruptcy proceedings. Seven had operated under involuntary receivers and seven under voluntary receivers
appointed by the Health Department. In the majority of cases in which
voluntary receivers have been appointed (those made at the request of the
operators), financial problems were the primary reason, while felony convictions against the operators were the reason for the appointment of most
of the involuntary receivers.

The frustration of enforcing standards is perhaps best illustrated by a
large nursing home in New York City. The owner, who was primarily
involved in construction of facilities, opened the facility in December 1973.
Immediately, complaints began to be lodged. Complaints alleged misuses of
personal funds and Social Security checks, inadequate feeding, lack of
medication, unanswered call bells, nursing service deficiencies, unsanitary

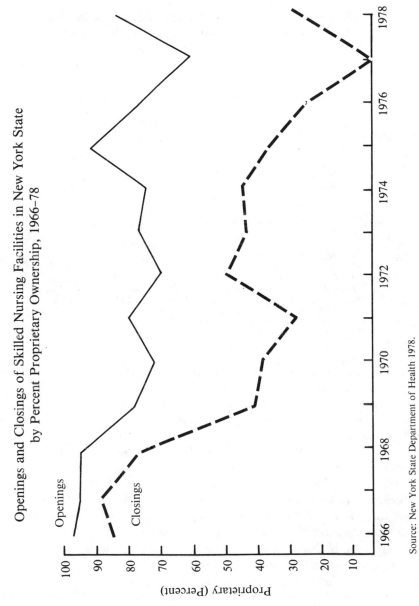

Figure 2.5

Openings and Closings of Skilled Nursing Facilities in New York State
by Percent Proprietary Ownership, 1966–78

Source: New York State Department of Health 1978.

Figure 2.6

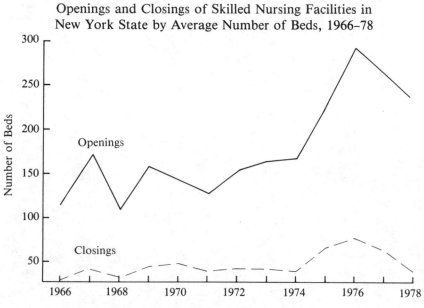

Openings and Closings of Skilled Nursing Facilities in
New York State by Average Number of Beds, 1966–78

Source: New York State Department of Health 1979.

food-handling, a patient who was discharged with pulmonary edema, gangrene and respiratory distress, excessive medication, the death of a patient from dehydration, rat and mice infestation, water bugs, inadequate heating, hot water that was too hot, complaints of a patient's throwing feces in a neighbor's yard, a shortage of blankets, and so on. Serious operating deficiencies were identified in July 1975 (Respondent 20 1978). In the summer of 1976, the Health Department took steps to impose fines and revoke the operator's license. Hearings began in September 1976. They proceeded at a leisurely pace, averaging about one a month. The process was further slowed by the operator's changing legal counsel several times during the proceedings. The appeals continued in spite of efforts on the part of the Health Department. The entire armamentarium of the Health Department was pitted against the facility: graduated fines, low reimbursement ratings, referral of criminal negligence charges to the Office of the Special Prosecutor, threatened withdrawal of federal Medicaid funding, and so on. All were effectively countered with legal maneuvering. Finally, on 13 February 1979, the operator's certificate was revoked and the Commissioner of Health was appointed as receiver, two and a half years after the hearings were begun.

It has proven cumbersome and extremely time-consuming to revoke an operator's license because of continuing violations of the Nursing Home Code. Certainly, no one could argue that these proceedings served to protect the patient from any "imminent danger to their health or safety."

Starting in January 1975, the orientation of the regional surveyors shifted from consultation to enforcement. Central office pressure was placed on the regional teams to identify facilities with significant deficiencies, undertake surprise inspections, and start exercising the ability to impose fines. A large number of deficiencies began to be identified, and relationships between the surveyor teams and the operators became increasingly strained. Survey teams were accused of "Gestapo tactics" and of gloating over the identification of weaknesses. Survey team members began to get pressure from both sides. There was pressure from Albany to develop an effective track record in terms of enforcement through imposition of fines and revocation of licenses. Efforts in this direction embroiled surveyors in time-consuming hearings for which they often felt ill-prepared.

Take, for example, the following cat-and-mouse exchange between a Health Department sanitarian and the attorney for a home in one of the graduated fine hearings. The deficiency cited had to do with corrosion in a dishwasher used by the home (New York State Department of Health 1978):

Q. All right, as to Charge No. 3, the dishwasher, your charge states that, or the letter sent out on June 3rd, Exhibit 3, it states, the dishwashing machine was not maintained in good repair, while the dishwasher appears to be providing proper wash and rinse temperatures and pressure, at the present time the machine is incurring more frequent repairs due to age and condition during our inspection. Was the machine performing properly?

A. It appeared to be performing properly.

Q. And the dishes that were cleaned were sanitary?

A. It appeared that they were clean and sanitary.

Q. So how would this affect or be a violation of the sanitary code?

A. The sanitary code called for the machine to be kept in good repair, as I stated, that there was a rug plugging up holes in the dishwashing machine, the outside was exhibiting corrosion, and stone buildup, especially on the vacuum breaker and the interior was exhibiting signs of a lime buildup.

Q. Would the lime buildup make the machine unsanitary?

A. It makes it harder to clean.

Q. Does it make it unsanitary?

A. If the machine cannot be properly cleaned, the machine becomes unsanitary.

Q. Yes, but when you found — when you inspected the machine, it was sanitary; correct?

A. (No response.)

Q. There is no violation listed for stating that it is unsanitary.

A. I have forgotten the beginning of his questioning.

Q. The charge does not state that the machine was unsanitary.

A. The charge says, should be in good repair.

Q. All right, you stated on your follow-up visit of July 5th, that you again checked the machine?

A. Yes.

Q. All right, were you shown an order for a machine at that time?

A. Yes, I was.

Q. Would the ordering of a machine have been in compliance, or would it have taken installation within 30 days to be compliance?

A. If there was the signature by the administrator as well as the monetary deposit put down on the machine and written on the order, then I would accept it as substantial progress.

Q. Did you ask anyone at the nursing home as to the expected date of delivery?

A. I cannot recall.

Q. Why would it be necessary to place a deposit on the purchase of a machine?

A. (No response.)

Q. To satisfy you that the order was completed?

A. Without a deposit down, it gives the facility the option to cancel the order without any penalty by the company who would be providing the product. With a deposit down, it shows intent, strong intent to purchase the dishwashing machine.

Q. Are you familiar with contract law?

A. No.

Q. But you are making a determination that a deposit is necessary?

(NYSDH, 1978a:25-30)

The lawyers would often attempt to demean and challenge the credibility of the witness. They asked questions about training and education. In one case involving a revocation hearing, the home's attorney proceeded to rub the ink from a marker used to label photographs submitted as evidence all over the picture and then protest: "What do you mean the photograph *clearly* shows the deficiency? It is all smudged (Respondent 44 1978)!"

Sometimes, however, the more aggressive tactics can backfire. Even the most high-powered, high-priced attorney who has succeeded in intimidating his witness can't afford to ignore the basic rule of never asking a question to which one doesn't know the answer (Respondent 44 1978):

> Attorney: What do you mean the tuna fish was prepared improperly?
>
> Witness: An obese, hairy, sweating, kitchen worker in an undershirt was mixing the tuna fish in a large pot. The tuna fish would get stuck in his armpits and then fall back in.

Major reorganization efforts began in 1977. The Health Department was divided into the traditional public health and health facility regulatory activities (standards enforcement, reimbursement, certificate of need). Those with legal or public finance backgrounds took over much of the public health physician's traditional leadership on the regulatory side. Area administrators, rather than regional public health physician commissioners, assumed control of the regional offices. The entire standards certification effort has undertaken a series of reorganizations that has served to emphasize the focus on enforcement, as opposed to simple professional consultation with operators. To many of the survey team members, this appeared to be a double message. The old concern with upgrading standards had been diluted with new concerns over efficiency. Added to the conflicting pressures on surveyors now embroiled in a tug-of-war between the industry and the Albany office are traumas related to efforts to dramatically reshape their role.

The 1976 cost control pressures brought the clear realization that the Health Department was working at cross-purposes. On the one hand, the standards certification group could not be documenting the need for additional staff and resources in order to upgrade facilities (thus justifying rate increases), while, on the other hand, regulatory efforts were being bent toward figuring out ways to reduce, or at least to freeze, reimbursement. Toward the end of 1976, there began to be a dramatic shift in the directives from Albany to the regional survey teams. The 1977 program plan for the Division of Health Facility Standards altered the focus away from the simple upgrading of standards [New York State Department of Health, Division of Health Facility Standards 1977 (italics added)]:

> The survey process should not generate cost incurring mandates or suggestions, unless absolutely necessary. The relationship between the surveillance program and costs resulting from overzealous enforcement must never be

ignored. *Reimbursement and enforcement are blood relatives, which should not and must not become estranged.* The costs of long-term care in New York must be significantly moderated now. Prudence in the survey process is essential to the moderation of costs.

To many surveyors this not only sounded like a reversal of earlier directives, it was tantamount to treason. Not only was the Albany office telling them essentially to back off, it was now reorganizing them into alien roles. A generalist inspection process was to replace the multidisciplinary team approach. Surveyors were to perform as generalists, as do surveyors in the majority of states. This would presumably entail savings in the survey effort itself as well as weaken the inflationary professional orientation of the New York survey process. Further, surveyors were now requested to perform management assessments, a process developed in response to a class action suit by the voluntary nursing homes concerning their rates for 1976. A makeshift, ad hoc process had developed to review the situation in each home and to determine if, in fact, the new reimbursement rates created serious problems from which the home needed financial relief. The surveyors were not only being asked to be generalists, but efficiency experts as well. Frustration within the regional survey staff reached a new peak.

A meeting was scheduled for 22–23 April 1977 to discuss the new generalist approach with all of the state surveyors. The commissioners who came to discuss the plan with the surveyors were greeted with booing and hissing. Concerned about the possible press coverage, the commissioners let the surveyors talk and simmer down, rather than discuss the details of the plan. They were faced with "tremendous hostility" (Respondent 41 1978).

The generalist approach struggled along for about a year. There were complaints from operators about the inconsistencies. Social work "generalist" surveyors in some cases continued to list primarily social work deficiencies. The program could not demonstrate any administrative efficiencies, and this, coupled with the continuing resistance of the surveyors themselves, led to its abandonment. At this point, the Office of Health Systems Management decided to make a new attempt to sort out the pieces by entering a $150,000 contract with an outside management consultant group to review the process and recommend changes.

The consultants systematically reviewed quality assurance, patient placement and assessment, utilization, and licensure and certification programs of the Health Department. The problems identified were similar to many of those reflected in this chapter. The detailed recommendations of the study are currently being reviewed and implemented by a series of Health Department task forces. The review of management assessment concluded that there was a great deal of confusion in the regional offices over implementation of the program, and that it did, as an earlier evaluation by the Division of the Budget had found, tend to be biased toward increased costs (Rensselaer Polytechnic Institute 1979, part 3, pp. 64–67). The major recommendations emphasized the need to better integrate and clarify the relationship between cost and quality and to develop far clearer guidelines and manuals for management assessment teams.

The management assessment process has been undergoing changes since its inception. The Division of the Budget study of the process, completed in the fall of 1978, was critical, as were those individuals who have been directly involved in the process. Management assessments were largely left up to the regional survey staff to complete, with relatively little guidance or training. They were to review patient mix and other possible explanations for divergence in financial needs of the institutions and to make recommendations; these, in turn, were forwarded to the Division of Long-Term Care Reimbursement to make the necessary adjustments in rates. The surveyors, sympathetic to the plight of the homes in their area and concerned about patient care, generally gave the institutions the benefit of the doubt. The Division of the Budget saw this as a gaping hole in the cost control program and was concerned with plugging the leak.

The Moreland Act Commission expressed dismay at the code that the surveyors used. As did the JCAH, it placed heavy emphasis on structural measures of care: that is, on whether what were professionally judged as necessary ingredients for good patient care existed. There was excessive emphasis on the paper documentation provided by the facility and relatively little on directly looking at patients and the care they were receiving. The Moreland Commission attempted to assess the validity of the process by comparing the results of such surveys with the Periodic Medical Reviews, which involve a review of each Medicaid patient's records and observations of the patient. A comparison of the PMR and the survey evaluations in a stratified sample of facilities revealed no significant correlations (Moreland Act Commission 1975). The Moreland Commission report, however, did indicate that higher reimbursement rates were positively correlated with fewer deficiencies identified in the survey. There was no significant positive correlation between level of reimbursement and adequacy of patient care, as judged by the Periodic Medical Reviews. Indeed, the only two significant correlations were negative (Moreland Act Commission 1975, p. 104). These results support the suspicions of the Division of Health Facilities Standards.

New York has not been alone in raising questions concerning the survey and certification process. At the federal level since 1974 there has been ongoing experimentation with more outcome-oriented methods of review. A series of patient data procedures designed both for planning patient care and for the assessment of outcomes have been developed and field tested by the Health Care Financing Administration's Division of Long-Term Care. One objective of these activities has been to identify a method for assessing quality of care that avoids the weaknesses of the indirect structural approach currently predominating in the survey and certification process. Hearings were conducted in 1978 by both the Health Standards and Quality Bureau and by the Senate subcommittee on federal spending practices and open government (U.S. Senate, 1978). The Bureau hearings resulted in consideration of a number of changes in the survey and certification process, the most significant being to assure greater consumer input and greater flexibility in the survey process. The Senate hearings voiced concerns about the "paper albatross" nature of the process similar to those expressed by most respondents in New York State (U.S., Senate, 1978).

Chapter 76 cost control legislation passed in the spring of 1976 created even greater pressure to review the State Nursing Home Code. The Health Department was neither enthusiastic nor optimistic about the implementation of these controls. The legislation called for the creation of minimum and maximum standards for licensure and for reimbursement tailored to meeting such standards. The rating system, initially viewed as a consumer tool, got tied into the new reimbursement scheme. Laying such a complex set of new requirements on top of the old nursing home code meant building on what most people had come to regard as a shaky foundation. Discussions with federal representatives concerning alteration of the code and standards had begun. In the fall of 1976, the Commissioner of Health pulled together a task force to work on developing a new code. The new code was to focus on performance and outcome in terms of patient care and eliminate the emphasis on paperwork, which was burdening both the operators and the Health Department. The task force was headed by George Warner, who had assisted in the development of the original code. He instructed those who participated in the process to "forget about the existing code, forget about the existing surveillance system, and start completely from scratch" (Respondent 9 1978). There was a concerted effort to break loose from traditional thinking about standards and enforcement. Participants were to explore all sources and strategies in terms of quality assurance, including the use of consumer ombudsmen, mail survey forms, Professional Standards Review Organizations, surveyors, and fire underwriters as sources of information concerning building fire safety. For guidelines, they were given a list of ten questions to which the process should provide answers (see Table 2.3).

The activities began with a small nucleus within the Health Department and expanded to include both the traditional interest groups and some new ones. Key regional field surveyors were canvassed. Both the facility associations and the professional associations were requested to submit a list of

Table 2.3

Guidelines for the Development of a New Code.

Questions to be asked of each hospital in New York State
to determine quality of services

1) Does the facility identify and profile the health care, environmental, and social support needs of each user prior to or at the time of admission, and periodically thereafter, in accordance with a plan of care that is modified promptly to meet changing needs of each user?

2) Does the facility provide services to match each user's needs; does it assess the extent to which each user's profiled needs are changed or the expected outcomes are achieved; and does the facility modify its services accordingly?

3) Does the facility provide a current and continuing analysis and evaluation of the profiled needs of its entire population of users and of the effective distribution and use of its resources and processes?

4) Does the facility efficiently provide and maintain a healthful, safe, and functional environment with environmental supports and safeguards matched to the needs of each user?

5) Does the facility deploy staff efficiently according to the qualifications and training of each; and [does the facility] utilize its support services efficiently relative to the profit of users' needs within the facility and in comparison to other providers of services for users with comparable needs?

6) Does the facility provide protection for the rights of all users and staff, and does each of its staff respect each user's rights to privacy and dignity?

7) Does the facility admit, retain, and provide services for its users without discrimination because of sex, race, creed, color, national origin, and source of payment?

8) Does the facility make available, as a matter of public record, information about its ownership, financial affairs, policies, and practices, exclusive of privileged or confidential information about individual users or staff?

9) Does the facility utilize its franchise (certificate of need) positively to meet community needs and to modify services as community needs change?

10) Does the facility coordinate its services with those of other providers of institutional and noninstitutional health and social services in the community through functioning affiliations and other mechanisms whereby the feasibility of meeting users' needs in other settings is periodically examined?

Source: New York State Department of Health, 1979.

individuals they felt were most expert in a particular area. Key professional staff from the Health Department picked five or six people from these lists to work with them in developing standards in a particular area. Public meetings were held in Rochester, Albany, and New York City in March and April of 1977. The first meeting in New York City proved tumultuous. The consumer groups viewed the meetings as a pro forma gesture on the part of the Health Department to legitimize an almost completed document. The failure of the Health Department to consult earlier with the Office of the Special Prosecutor, which had attempted to work closely with the consumer groups in New York City, fueled suspicions. Both the Office of the Special Prosecutor and the New York City consumer groups (Friends and Relative of the Institutionalized Aged, Legal Services for the Elderly Poor, and so on) became actively involved in the process of developing a new code. One of the lessons of the past, from the point of view of the Health Department, was to make sure that, this time, the process would be an open one. If it had not been so before the April 1977 meeting, it became so then.

Something happened in the process. The code became more specific. Paperwork was not reduced in most areas, and, in some areas related to patient rights, it increased dramatically. There was less flexibility in the new code than in the original. Although somewhat more focused on patient care, it was more oriented toward procedure and placed less reliance on clinical judgments of outcome than did the prior code.

No one was particularly happy with the outcome. At a second meeting held in New York City later in the year, Health Department officials could get some satisfaction from their new role as arbitrator between the consumer and provider groups, rather than as the focus of hostility. There were heated exchanges between operators, consumer group representatives, the Office of the Special Prosecutor, and the Health Department, particularly concerning the patients' rights sections. The climate was not right for performance-oriented standards that rely on professional judgment. The public's deep distrust of providers and the regulatory apparatus, particularly in New York City, continued to be reinforced with cases of nursing home abuse. The inability of the Health Department to quickly close facilities helped demonstrate the weakness of the more subjective elements of the old code. The Palatine decision sealed its fate. In an adversary environment, where there is pervasive distrust of both operators and regulators, the professional model of control ceases to be a meaningful alternative.

It was not until late in the 1978 legislative session that it became apparent that, in order to implement the new code, legislation would have to be passed eliminating the mini-maxi requirements created in the 1976 legislation. Without realizing the implications, the task force had been revising the state standards (part 700 maxi standards). Facilities, as a result of the 1976 legislation, are required to comply only with the federal standards (part 400 mini standards). Thus, without legislative repeal of the mini-maxi provisions, the new code was unenforceable. That legislative repeal was not enacted. There was a feeling in the legislature that the Health Department had not earnestly attempted to implement the mini-maxi system or the system of tying reimbursement to rating. Industry association representatives were also active in pointing out the potential cost of the new code, variously estimated at an additional $20 to $200 million. After the investment of energy and idealism, drafts and redrafts, and the involvement of over one hundred people, the new code was left, at least in the short run, to twist slowly in the wind.

The Health Department, however, appears to be making some progress toward sorting through all of the problems related to the surveillance program.

In 1979 a $150,000 contract with a research group produced a comprehensive assessment of the program and made recommendations that are in the process of being implemented. That study picked up on most of the issues identified in this chapter.

A project implementation team has been established in the Health Department, including a long-term care coordinator from one of the regional offices, a lawyer, a personnel expert, and an individual from the Health Department standards group. An elaborate, phased implementation strategy is being completed. Possible bottlenecks include (i) waiver of federal regulatory requirements from the Health Care Financing Administration, (ii) elimination of the existing rating legislation, and (iii) elimination of the mini-maxi legislation. These activities are aimed at clearing away the accumulated underbrush and developing a logical, understandable process of surveillance. This process includes:

1) Elimination of duplicate items from the various survey requirements.

2) Self-documentation by the facility of about half of the remaining 250 items in the combined survey document. (Surveyors will conduct some sample validation of these items, with potential sanctions for fraudulent completion by operators.)

3) A screening survey by inspectors designed to satisfy the remainder of the sixteen federal conditions of Medicare and Medicaid participation. There are conditions of participation under these programs, which, in turn, are broken down into 96 standards and, even finer, into 525 elements of care. The screening survey would focus on the standard level and not be designed to review every single element of care.

4) Simultaneously with the standard survey, an outcome-oriented

Periodic Medical Review of all patients would be completed. This would focus on sentinel health events, or generally recognized signals of potential problems in quality of care (for example indwelling catheters, restraints, bedsores, transfers within, transfers out, falls and accidents, infections, and mortality). A checklist of sentinel health events would be used to review each patient. Norms would be established and used to signal potential problems. If the norms were exceeded, an in-depth process review of a sample of patients would be undertaken. Protocols would be developed to guide such a review and assure consistency throughout the system. Pass-fail criteria related to each protocol would be used to determine the necessity of a deficiency report.

5) The results from the screening survey and the Periodic Medical Reviews and process reviews would be used to determine if a more intensive survey were necessary.

6) Should a more intensive survey be necessary, it would be carried out by a special team of surveyors specifically trained to deal with problem facilities and enforcement problems.

7) A validation team from the central office will do surprise inspections of facilities to assure uniformity of enforcement and reduce the ability of facilities to predict the timing of their next inspection.

The process as it is currently being conceptualized is summarized by the flow chart in Figure 2.7. Normally, the external inspection process for health facilities follows a deductive logic which assumes that, if the paperwork and physical structure meet acceptable standards, appropriate process quality and patient care outcomes will follow. The proposed inspection process reverses this order, at least partially, and focuses first on patient care outcomes and then on failings of individuals or structure that can account for it. Professionals are perhaps excessively concerned with structure and process outcome. The approach is refreshing in that it is coherent, avoids the cumulative mindlessness that others have unsuccessfully struggled against, and seems to effectively address the criticism of a lack of attention to actual patient care. Inspectors recently received several days of intensive training at the state police barracks on investigatory techniques and interrogation of witnesses, perhaps in an attempt to further alter this mind set. The changes will no doubt meet with resistance from some consumer groups who suspect that increased flexibility implies a watering down of standards. Operators and, possibly, inspection personnel may be a little too scared and weary to embrace the changes immediately or with much enthusiasm. Whether these changes will be any more effective in untying the Gordian knot of enforcement remains to be seen. In February 1980 a report

Figure 2.7

Proposed Review Process for Long-Term Care Facilities

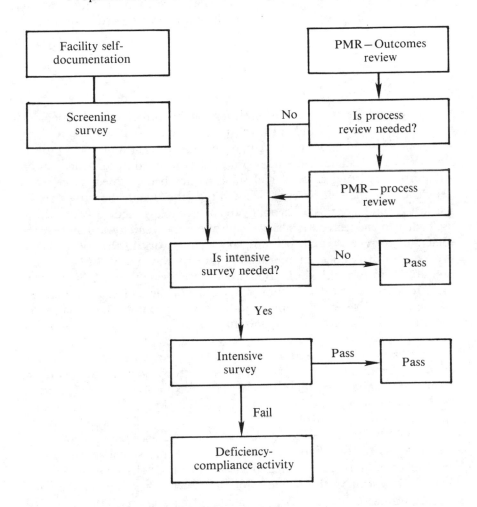

Source: New York State Department of Health 1979.

of an internal investigation within the Health Department documented the continuing existence of shocking neglect of patients in some homes and the continued inability to punish operators who allowed such conditions to exist (NYSDH). The refinements in the survey process had yet to be implemented by mid-1980. The frustration of enforcing standards, illustrated by the New York experience, is mirrored in other states which have faced similar administrative and legal problems in their attempts to establish stricter enforcement.

Conclusions

This review of efforts to tighten professional controls on nursing homes in New York State is a study of frustration. In spite of efforts to refine the survey process and make it a more rigorous enforcement tool, it has proven slow and cumbersome. The survey process has resulted in some licenses of administrators being revoked and some homes being closed, largely for deficiencies in the Life Safety Code. On the other hand, the survey effort has lost ground in terms of its ability to enforce many sections of the existing code. No one feels particularly happy about the trend toward more specificity, more rigidity, and, perhaps, more paperwork in the code-making process, but there does not appear to be an easy way out of the bind. Current efforts to refine the inspection process are trying to make the process more reasonable, but they cannot escape most of the underlying problems. At the heart of the process appear to be some basic dilemmas concerning professional controls and the organization of an extremely complex federal-state regulatory effort.

The frustrations expressed by respondents appear to be variations on the theme of professional controls in the health sector in general. Similar complaints are raised concerning the JCAH accreditation process (Johnson 1977). The ideal in professional control, salaried physicians in practice who share responsiblity for quality of care, appears to suffer from similar problems (Freidson 1975). Extreme cases of incompetence or negligence are eventually rooted out, but it is a slow process. Professional control essentially relies on normative power: that is, individuals share values and are motivated to achieve those values for their own sakes and for the good opinion of their colleagues. Education and persuasion are all that is needed to achieve compliance. When those shared values do not exist, however, the structure tumbles like a house of cards. This is the first side of the professional control dilemma: how to deal with the deviant without undermining the shared values and collegial relationships of the majority. The other side of the dilemma is how to control those professional values themselves.

Half of the inflation in health care costs in the last ten years has been the result of improved standards and new technology. Beginning in 1976, New York faced this dilemma of rising expectations in terms of standards and rising concerns about cost. This in essence is what the surveyors had to deal with. They were told to improve the standards of care but avoid recommendations that would serve to justify additional reimbursement. The roles of policeman and efficiency expert were added to that of professional consultant. The Office of Health Systems Management, however, had great difficulty in enforcing this shift in orientation on their field staffs.

This ambivalence and the resulting confusion is heightened by the nature of the regulatory machinery. Figure 2.8 illustrates the flow of influences on inspection efforts, including federal legislative and administrative initiatives, development of federal regulations, regional HHS interpretation and implementation, state legislative and administrative initiatives, Health Department interpretation and implementation, operator reaction in terms of acceptance or administrative and legal appeals, and, in some cases, court decisions concerning the legality of the regulations. The process takes at least three or four years to work through. In the case of the Life Safety Code enforcement, it took close to ten years. In the interim, administrations change, new legislation is passed, and the emphasis shifts. In such a process, a regulator does not embrace too quickly or invest too much ego in any new initiative.

As a result, the regulator, no matter where he fits into the process, sees himself as besieged. He has sweeping and constantly changing responsibilities. He faces a well-organized industry, a legal system concerned about the protection of property rights, and a legislature that finds "bureaucrats" safe targets for ridicule and whose rhetoric of concern is rarely matched either by depth of understanding or the necessary appropriations.

Above all, the regulator must engage in intense parochial rivalries with the various state and federal bureaus, divisions, and agencies and the voluntary professional groups with whom he shares responsibility for the assurance of standards. It is an environment that does not reward innovation. It encourages ritualized responses to guidelines. Innovation invites harassment from other regulators or from the industry. If one makes sure to protect oneself on paper (that is, if one essentially does not try), one cannot be faulted for the failure. Regulators feel the same pressures toward ritualistic behavior that they impose on the homes they regulate. It is understandable, then, that innovations such as more flexible, selective surveillance have been slow in being implemented.

There are other, more subtle pressures that weaken the rigor of the surveillance process. First, state agencies involved in such processes are usually part of a larger structure that is responsible for setting rates, approving

Figure 2.8

The Ebb and Flow of Health Care
Standard Regulations

Interest Group Activities ———————▶ *Passage of Federal Legislation*

General public relations
Focused lobbying of key legislators and
  committee staff and administrative agencies
Legal action against federal and state agencies
  responsible for implementing intent of
  legislation

Introduction of bill in House or Senate
Referral to committee for study
Referral to subcommittee for hearings, revision,
  and recommendations
Report to full committee
Floor action
Conference committee action:
  resolution of any differences in House and
  Senate version of bill
Presidential approval (or veto and legislative
  override) producing public law requiring a
  federal agency to develop regulations to
  comply with the intent of the legislation

STATE AND FEDERAL
COURTS

State Agency Implementation of ◀——————— *Department of Health, Education, and Welfare*
Intent of Legislation   *Implementation of Intent of Legislation*

State agency reviews and clarifies rules
Transmittal to subcontracting state or municipal
  agency
Transmittal to Regional health department office
  of area administrator
Review and training sessions with Medicaid
  standard program supervisor and inspection
  staff
Survey teams implement requirements
Institutional resistance
Requests of state and regional federal agency
  for clarification

Announcement in *Federal Register* of rule-
  making intent, providing opportunity for
  interested parties to participate through
  submission of views
Publication of drafted rules in *Federal Register,*
  providing further opportunity for review and
  comment
Public hearings and submission of written
  comments
Final rules published in *Federal Register,* rules
  become incorporated in *Code of Federal
  Regulations*
Agency central office prepares transmittal of
  regional office

licensure of facilities, and determining the issues of cost, quality, and access to health services. Reports of inadequate care by the standard surveillance branch reflect poorly on its sister bureaus. In New York, as in other states, there has been a continuing effort to better integrate these functions. This integration may increse efficiency and reduce overt conflicts. Whether it will affect the willingness to identify significant deficiencies, however, remains to be seen.

Second, the surveyors themselves are caught between increasingly divided loyalties to their agency and their institutions. Surveyors are not rotated from one region to another, as a matter of policy, as are state policemen. This rotation is designed to assure uniformity of performance and loyalty to the central organization. Many religious denominations rotate their clergy for similar reasons.

Finally, the outcomes of inspection of facilities are subject to review, but that review process focuses largely upon the possibility of what in statistics are called Type I errors, or false positives. That is, the agency may mistakenly cite a facility or take other action against it for substandard care. An elaborate administrative and judicial review process will follow in almost every case where the decision adversely affects the home.

As a result, every report of a significant operating deficiency is reviewed by at least five levels within the Health Department before a notice is sent to the facility. On the other hand, what in statistics are called Type II errors, or false negatives (that is, the surveyor passes a facility that has serious operational deficiencies), could easily go unnoticed. In the past, such cases were not even subjected to sample reliability checks by validation survey teams. Although procedures have now been implemented in New York to perform such checks, the judgments of the surveyors are not subjected to the same intense scrutiny as are reports of observed operating deficiencies.

Other things being equal, these pressures will tend to erode the willingness of the agency and of the individual surveyor to more rigorously enforce operating standards and will lead them toward more ritualized processing. There are limits, therefore, to what the existing process of professional standards enforcement can achieve. The next chapter will review the effectiveness of reimbursement incentives for both cost and quality control.

Chapter Three

Tightening Fiscal Controls

"Money doesn't talk, it swears" — Bob Dylan

Reimbursement shapes the system. That unrelenting force builds, destroys, distorts, corrupts, and sometimes actualizes dreams. The self-styled social architect might wish to create an ideal system of delivery and then, as an afterthought, create a reimbursement system to support it. In reality, the system is constructed around reimbursement. These mechanisms have been an historical accumulation, a patchwork that must be stitched together into an often irrational, costly, and sometimes dehumanizing pattern.

Given reimbursement's power for both creating and destroying, it was only natural that, in the wake of the New York State nursing home scandals, increased interest would be focused on this area. How can the system of payment to nursing homes be altered to better avoid abuse and to control costs? How can it be used to provide incentives for higher quality care? The first question involves refining the method of reimbursement, tightening the administration and control of the program. On the surface this appeared to be a fairly straightforward task. However, as will be described in this chapter, controlling an appropriate flow of public funds to nursing homes was fraught with difficulties.

The second question, how to create financial incentives for higher quality care, involved an ill-equipped voyage into uncharted waters that foundered on both methodological and philosophical rocks.

Before the passage of Medicare and Medicaid in 1965, responsibility for providing nursing home care for the indigent was shared by state and local governments.

The enactment of Medicaid in 1965 did not, in itself, represent a radical break with the past in terms of the pattern of financing care for the indigent elderly. Nor are the current concerns with the cost of such a program of recent origin. Indeed, the first public concern about the rising cost of such care in New York State dates back to at least the 1820s. [The cost of caring for the indigent rose from $245,000 in 1815 to $475,000 in 1822, not quite equalling more recent rates of increase in Medicaid costs (Thomas 1969, p. 17).] Concern about these costs to both the state and local governments led to an emphasis on indoor relief, county poor farms and workhouses, rather than direct subsidies. Direct subsidies were felt to be too costly to administer and too tempting. It was felt that, if conditions for relief were made sufficiently unpleasant, the indolent would not be tempted. Over the next century, public interest fluctuated between concern over costs and concern over the conditions in these facilities, a phenomenon similar to fluctuating concerns over the Medicaid program. Reforms prohibited children (in 1875) and the mentally ill (in 1890) from being placed in these facilities. There was a growing revulsion against indoor relief. The State Charities Aid Association, which had established visiting committees in every county and had the legal right to inspect any poor house after 1881, did much to expose conditions. A national study in the 1920s exposing conditions in poor farms got widespread attention (Thomas 1969, pp. 24–36).

The New York State Old Age Security Act of 1930 specifically prohibited support to elderly in institutions, in order to avoid the stigma of associating this program with the poor farms. The federal Social Security Act, modeled after the New York legislation, followed suit, with similar prohibitions in terms of the aged and the blind.

As is so often the case in public policy, the rhetoric and images that guided the Social Security legislation had not kept pace with the realities. Reform efforts, demographic shifts, and industrialization had gradually transformed these institutions into ones caring for older, sicker individuals who were less capable of taking care of themselves. County welfare commissioners were faced with the task of finding places to put these people.

One major concern of local commissioners was the local cost of the welfare program. These costs could be reduced by placing their wards in private homes, where they would be eligible for Old Age Assistance, rather than in the large public and voluntary facilities. Thus, the proprietary nursing home sector emerged. As indicated in Figure 3.1, the number of facilities grew rapidly, while the number of public and voluntary nursing home beds remained relatively static until the mid-1960s. As support for the elderly indigent grew, the proprietary nursing home sector grew. The wood frame residences accommodating fewer than a dozen individuals began to be replaced by larger, more medically-oriented facilities.

County welfare commissioners negotiated contracts with the homes for the care of welfare patients. The contracts were established on the basis of

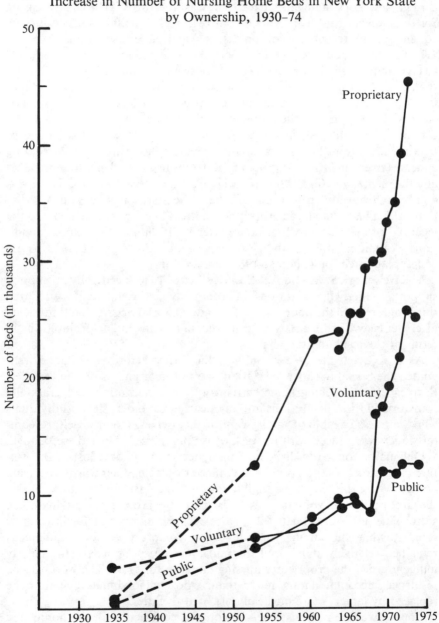

Figure 3.1

Increase in Number of Nursing Home Beds in New York State
by Ownership, 1930–74

Source: Thomas 1969 for 1935–64; Dunlop 1979 for 1964–74.

per diem charges rather than costs. The charges were the subject of negotiation between the local commissioner and the homes. This was done individually or collectively, depending on the locality. The charge was based on the willingness of the commissioner to pay and the willingness of the home to accept welfare patients at that price.

Negotiations in New York City developed more sophistication than did those in other areas of the state. The Metropolitan Nursing Home Association negotiated with the New York City Commissioner of Welfare a uniform charge-based rate for all proprietary homes in the City. Independently audited uniform cost reports were required of all homes by the commissioner beginning in 1962. These, however, were not used in determining rates, but in facilitating informed negotiations with the homes. At about the same time, the Metropolitan Nursing Home Association began to negotiate for its members with unions, and to sponsor continuing education programs.

The major impetus for the greater collaboration among the proprietary nursing homes in New York City appears to have come from investigations initiated by the City Department of Investigations in 1958. A probe of eighty-eight proprietary homes in the City alleged shocking conditions and padded payrolls. The Heyman Commission, headed by Ray Trussell, made a series of recommendations. Inspectors were added, whereas there had been no increase in their number in the City between 1930 and 1955 (Thomas 1969, p. 195). Even some night inspections were carried out. A new City code for nursing homes was developed with the assistance of eighty committee people and a small grant from a foundation. The code was considered the most strict in the nation and was later to be used in developing a uniform state code (Respondent 9 1978).

One unintended outcome of these efforts toward stricter regulation was a more unified, disciplined, and sophisticated proprietary association. The current offensive appears to have had a similar impact on all of the associations representing nursing home interests.

The essentially charge-based rates before 1966 had two implications for the exposés that were to follow ten years later. First, since reimbursement was based on an agreed-upon charge rather than directly tied to the cost of providing services, the opportunities for fraud by operators were more limited. The operator's per diem charge was essentially his to do with as he saw fit, as long as he met local health department standards. It was not directly tied to the various components of care. The change to a cost-based statewide rate system in 1966 and its implications in terms of audit requirements were not universally appreciated until almost ten years later. Second, charge-based reimbursement essentially froze care within nursing homes: it provided no incentive for an operator to improve or expand services. It was tied to local welfare budgets and the reluctance of local governments to absorb increasing costs. Most facilities were wood frame buildings that were not fire-resistant. Training for nursing home administrators was non-existent. Registered nurses were often in short supply and sometimes non-existent. Few of the proprietary homes had social or rehabilitation services, now universally required.

The freeze, or at least stagnation, in development of nursing home standards ended with the passage of Article 28 and the enactment of Medicare and Medicaid in 1965. Governor Rockefeller had appointed the Committee on Hospital Costs in 1964 in response to public outcry to dramatic rises in Blue Cross rates. Marion Folsom, an Eastman Kodak executive and former secretary of HEW, who had also influenced the New York and federal Social Security legislation in the 1930s, served as chairman of the committee. The resulting legislation, Article 28, produced a dramatic shift in the locus, extent, and complexity of public regulatory activity. The state Health Department assumed responsibility for the development and enforcement of standards in all health care facilities and for the establishment of rates of reimbursement for both public assistance patients and for Blue Cross plans. The Metcalf-McCloskey Act, which had become law a year earlier, gave the Health Department the authority to license new facilities on the basis of demonstrated public need, the character and competence of operators, financial viability, and other matters within its discretionary powers. Thus, New York had developed a statewide certificate-of-need and planning apparatus, a rate-setting structure, and a standard-setting apparatus well in advance of other states' efforts.

The method of reimbursing nursing homes, however, had lagged behind hospital regulation in New York. Blue Cross plans in the state had begun to develop cost-related contracts with hospitals in the 1940s. The dramatic transformation of technology, manpower, and costs was attributable to this development as well as to the activities of the American College of Surgeons and, later, the JCAH. It is ironic that concern for the rising cost of hospital care triggered a similar transformation in nursing homes within the state. The new cost-based rate-setting mechanisms were taken out of the hands of the local social service commissioners. While local governments were required, under the Medicaid program as adopted by New York State, to contribute 25 percent of the cost, they were also required to make payments to homes on the basis of rates determined by the Health Department in Albany.

The impact of these decisions was not felt immediately. In the first year of fully cost-based rates, 1967, the actual rates certified by the Health Department were actually lower in 50 percent of the cases than were the rates negotiated by local commissioners in 1966 (Respondent 47 1979). This, however, was largely the result of the use of cost reports, which had not been collected for determining reimbursement. Providers reacted quickly to these changed conditions, and costs increased rapidly.

The counties soon became unable to meet their responsibilities in the financing of the Medicaid program. One of the eligibility criteria New York had adopted for the program was an annual income of $6,000 for a family of four, making a large portion of the population eligible. Increases in nursing home costs were exacerbated by the rapid disengagement of the federal Medicare program from the provision of nursing home services. This created a financial crisis for local government. Local Medicaid costs were more than double what was expected, and they resulted in large local tax increases. In 1968 the state legislature froze rates. A more detailed strategy for cost control was enacted later the same year, with relatively little input from either the hospital or nursing home associations. Article 28 of the Public Health Law was amended to require that rates be reasonably related to the costs of "efficient production of services." The Commissioner of Health was required to consider, in making such certification, (i) the elements of costs, (ii) geographic differentials in costs, (iii) economic factors in the area where the facility was, (iv) the rate of increase or decrease of the economy in the area, (v) costs of institutions of comparable size, and (vi) the need for incentives to improve services and institute economies. The legislation no longer allowed research and education costs. Rates calculated to comply with this legislation were established in January 1970. Some of the potential for profit in proprietary operations was also eliminated. Allowances for development, which most operators considered as profit, were discontinued, and an allowance for return of capital as a percentage of gross costs was replaced by a return of capital based on a percentage of the actual capital invested. Since then, the formula has been changed almost yearly. The economic stabilization program in 1972 brought additional restrictions. Throughout this period, hospitals seemed more capable of getting relief from the changing rate formulas than did nursing homes. In 1968 hospitals had a freeze imposed by the Health Department overturned by court action on the basis of federal Medicaid requirements for reasonable cost reimbursement for acute care. The freeze remained in effect for nursing homes. Similarly, in 1973, hospitals, also through court action, obtained relief from some of the limitations on cost increases imposed by the economic stabilization program, but the Health Department held in place the same limitations for nursing homes.

Thus, prior to 1974, nursing homes faced a centralized, sophisticated system of reimbursement that had gone through continuous refinements. New York State's nursing home reimbursement system was looked to as a model by other states faced with the federal requirements (P.L. 92–602,

Sec. 249, Oct. 30, 1972) of using a cost-based system of nursing home reimbursement for Medicaid recipients. (The states were faced with a 1 July 1976
deadline for implementing such a system. This deadline was later changed
to 1 January 1978). At that time, New York appeared to be the only state
that met the new requirements; thus, financial control problems New York
faced were of more widespread significance. The general prospective reimbursement approach continues to be advocated by many as the most appropriate means for controlling rising hospital costs. In order to understand the
hidden flaws, however, it is necessary to review the mechanics.

The increasingly sophisticated, constantly changing methods of rate calculation left all but those directly and immediately involved mystified. A
cat-and-mouse game evolved between the state and the nursing home industry from 1967 onward. The industry would identify loopholes, and the state
would make incremental adjustments designed to plug them (Spitz 1979, p.
33). The general pattern will only be summarized here, since a more detailed
description would have only transitory relevance.

The foundation for rate calculation is the cost report that must be filed by
facilities by the end of April for the previous calendar year (the reporting
requirements have increased over time). The reports must be certified by an
independent auditor. A desk review of the reports was performed by the
Health Department. Before 1975 reviews were generally performed conser-
vatively, since the Health Department had limited field audit capability. It
was felt that the institution could always appeal if improper disallowances
were made.

The system for calculating rates as of 1 January 1975 was summarized by
the Temporary State Commission on Living Costs and the Economy in the
flow chart that appears in Figure 3.2.

Real property costs and administrators' salaries were subject to ceilings
established by the Division of Health Economics. Administrative, dietary,
and housekeeping costs, combined, were subject to a cost ceiling of 10
percent above the peer group cost average. Peer groups were established on
the basis of size, geographic region, and type of ownership. For comparison
purposes and for determination of reimbursement to facilities, the total
number of patient days in 1973 was divided into costs to obtain a per diem
rate for both the peer group and the individual institution. Finally, an overall ceiling was determined by adding all costs in the peer group and dividing
by the total number of patient days—any costs 15 percent above this average were disallowed. Added to allowable per diem operating expenses were
(i) an inflation factor for increases in a health-service-related price index
over the two-year period, (ii) a return on equity, based on the Medicare rate
of return (10 percent in 1974), (iii) allowable capital per diem costs, and (iv)
for the provider whose costs were below the peer group average in adminis-

Figure 3.2

Calculations of Medicaid Reimbursement as of January 1, 1975

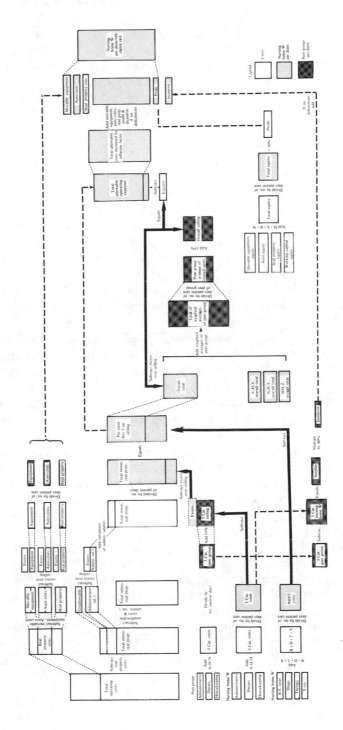

Source: Temporary State commission on Living Costs and the Economy (New York) 1975. p.83

trative, dietary, and housekeeping services, an efficiency incentive equal to 40 percent of the difference between his costs and the average costs. The outcome of this process, which began with the desk reviews, was a per diem rate that was routinely approved by the Division of the Budget and sent to county Social Services Department commissioners in a schedule of daily rates for each nursing home; commissioners were required to use the schedule in paying bills submitted to them by the homes for Medicaid patients.

The 1975 rate-setting formula was the result of nine years of refinement aimed at eliminating loopholes and creating greater efficiency within the industry. In spite of these efforts, costs rose between 1966 and 1975 from an average skilled nursing facility per diem of $13.00 to $37.09 (Moreland Act Commission 1976c, p. 140). Two significant factors entered into these increased costs besides health care wage catch-ups to general wage levels and inflation. First, the period involved a dramatic upgrading of standards, with increased staff and expanded programs reflected in changes in rates. Second, a capital building program began, with smaller homes replaced by larger fire-resistant facilities costing as much as $30,000 per bed; resulting increases in costs per day were as much as six or seven dollars (Moreland Act Commission 1976c, p. 141).

Underlying these cost increases in the industry was the relationship between the fiscal and the program sides of the Health Department. Generally, the program side was in the driver's seat. If the surveyors recommended increases in a home's rate in order to accommodate improvements they felt were necessary, and if the fiscal side felt convinced that this was not the result of gaming the prospective reimbursement system by the operator, those increases were generally honored.*

The prospective reimbursement methodology in itself did not appear to stem cost increases. It failed to escape the inflationary psychology of cost reimbursement because it was essentially based on a delayed-cost reimbursement. The potential controls of peer group cost ceilings were far less credible with nursing homes than with hospitals, since many peer group institutions had overlapping ownership.

The complexity of the rate calculation process perhaps helped to conceal the lack of auditing capability. As the Moreland Commission pointed out, any cost-reimbursed reporting mechanism that lacks audit capability or sanctions creates "an invitation to theft" (Moreland Act Commission 1976,

---

*One strategy that some operators attempted to use was to (i) lay off nursing staff in year T, (ii) pocket the reimbursements in year T that were based on costs and staffing levels in year T-2, and (iii) appeal in year T + 2 for reimbursement (initially based on costs and staffing in year T) to cover added nursing staff that Health Department surveyors determined were needed.

p. iv). This, according to interviews, was widely understood within both the proprietary and the voluntary sectors of the industry. According to one Nursing Home Association spokesperson, Association leadership had requested Health Department field audits as early as 1971 (Respondent 74 1978). Prior to 1971 there had been only one person available for field audits of all 625 nursing homes, 150 health-related facilities, 354 hospitals, 300 clinics, 120 home health agencies, 8 Article 9C corporations, and 6 health maintenance organizations. Only seventeen field audits of nursing homes had been completed between August 1968 and March 1971. Requests to the Division of the Budget for additional audit staff, however, continued to be turned down. As a result, there were abuses. These will be described in more detail in Chapter Four.

Perhaps by far the most potentially profitable avenue for abuse was in construction and sale of homes. Property costs were reimbursable within certain ceilings developed by the Division of Health Economics. There were instances of substantial profits by contractors. There were also fraudulently inflated building costs of operators who served as their own contractors, a practice not allowed by the regulations. In some cases, interlocking ownership of construction firms and nursing homes created abuse similar to the kickback arrangements with suppliers.

There were some exaggerated claims at the beginning of the scandals of rapid bogus sales and resales to increase capital reimbursement; these were not borne out by closer examination. A review of sales of proprietary homes from September 1971 to September 1974 identified only nine instances in which the sales resulted in a change of capital cost reimbursement. In only seven of these cases did reimbursement for capital costs increase (Moreland Act Commission 1976a, p. 137). Some such abuses, of course, may have occurred before 1971. A construction firm with no interest in operating a nursing home would still have to apply for a license under certificate-of-need legislation. A potential purchaser would be unlikely to buy without seeing at least detailed architectural drawings. The development of such costly detailed plans without first obtaining approval of the Public Health Council is inconceivable. Thus, construction firms that had no intention of operating a facility could be labeled "traffickers." That is not to say that such activities could not be extremely profitable. The construction firm or contractor-operator had obtained a franchise that provided a guaranteed income. Such a franchise was highly valued and aggressively sought. Most of the accusations of bribery and influence-peddling that grew out of the investigations focused on such efforts at obtaining operating certificates. Thus, a major focus of the reimbursement reforms was to control abuse of property cost reimbursement.

Changes

The fiscal controls that began to be imposed on nursing homes in 1975 were the result of provisions in the package of legislative proposals on nursing homes, and the subsequent Medicaid legislation and corresponding changes in the administration of the reimbursement program.

Administrative Changes

A series of organizational changes began to take place in the administration of the reimbursement program.

First, the Bureau of Audits and Investigations began to get the staff it had been requesting since its inception in 1971. Before then, there had been only one auditor in the Health Department available for field audits. From a staff of eight in early 1975, the Bureau grew to 167 auditors by the end of 1978. The regional organization of the Bureau of Audits and Investigations mirrors that of the Health Department as a whole. Each regional office has a team of auditors responsible for investigations in that region. The extensive audit programs that were devised involved on-site reviews that often lasted more than two months.

Second, larger organizational changes began to take place in 1977. The Division of the Budget took an active role in restructuring the regulatory activities and making sure operations, as they viewed them, "did not return to business as usual" (Respondent 54 1978). First, the regulatory functions were separated from the traditional Health Department functions into two offices, the Office of Health Systems Management and the Office of Public Health. The new structure replaced regional physician commissioners with area administrators. There was a dramatic shift in the leadership (described as purge by some respondents) away from the traditional public health professionals toward those with legal, financial, or managerial backgrounds. The new structure, still evolving, is outlined in Figure 3.3. Among its refinements was a Bureau of Residential Health Care Facilities Reimbursement, which has now assumed responsibility for capital as well as operating cost reimbursement. The specific changes that were set in motion by these efforts focused on control of abuse, control of cost increases, and the linkage of reimbursement to quality of care.

Legislative Reforms

The 1975 legislation included the following provisions aimed at controlling abuse within the long-term care reimbursement program:

1. Liability of controlling persons (Chapter 651) — Any person who

Figure 3.3

Organizational Chart of the New York State Department of Health

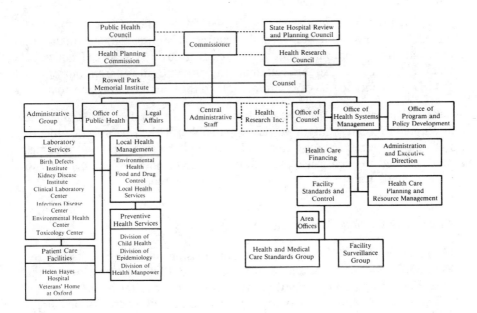

Source: Department of Health 1980.

directly or indirectly has the power to make policy or direct the management of the institution is liable for damages and civil penalties to the same extent that the facility is liable.

2. Report of ownership patterns in annual financial report (Chapter 652) — The report must identify the operator and anyone who holds a ten percent or greater interest in the land, building, or mortgage. Any interest of a lessor or lessee must be reported, as well an any transactions with any of the above individuals aggregating to $500 or more within the fiscal year.

3. Penalties for false financial statements (Chapter 659) — Fraudulently attempting to obtain payment from public funds for services or supplies for services furnished in connection with Medicaid reimbursement is a felony. In addition, local social service districts or the state may recover treble damages for false statements.

4. Criteria for reimbursement (Chapter 649) — The Commissioner of Health must develop a rate formula relating reimbursement to quality of care and linking reimbursement to the "prudent buyer" concept. That is, the Health Department should attempt to simulate in its reimbursement criteria payments for services comparable to those in a competitive market.

In summary, the fiscal control portions of this legislative package attempted to assure that all parties responsible for the operation be identified, that penalties for false financial statements be stiff, and that the rates be calculated in such a way as to increase the incentives for operators to bargain hard for the goods and services they purchased for care of their patients.

Changes in Capital Cost Reimbursement

The work of the Temporary State Commission on Living Costs and the Economy and the Moreland Commission had focused attention on the potential for abuse in terms of reimbursement for capital costs.

The issue of capital cost reimbursement had received continuous attention since the inception of New York's Medicaid program. For newly constructed facilities, a method similar to Medicare's capital cost reimbursement system was adopted. For older, converted facilities, an imputed rental system was developed. This was calculated on the basis of a percentage of leases or rentals that existed prior to the creation of the Medicaid program. It was believed that the charge-based reimbursement that existed before the Medicaid program would encourage hard bargaining by an operator. An inflation factor was added to these earlier leases to obtain the current imputed rental.

The Public Health Council was required to approve new facilities on the basis of the character and competence of the owners, financial feasibility, and public need. Any transfers of ownership had to be approved by the council. Attention was focused on capital cost reimbursement issues by the sale of one home that inflated actual costs by several million dollars. Investigations by an ad hoc committee on capital cost reimbursement of the council became the source for some *New York Times* articles by John Hess in the fall of 1974. The ad hoc committee's recommendations were adopted by the Health Department in March 1975, were replaced by those of the Moreland Commission in 1976 and 1977, and then were replaced by those of a joint executive-legislative task force for residential health care facilities' Medicaid reimbursement in January 1978. At the heart of these final changes, which had been approximated by earlier refinements, was a reassessment of the peculiar nature of property in this industry. The market value of property was largely attributable to the institution's franchise and the cost-related reimbursement that the franchise entitled it to receive. Successive efforts to alter methods of capital reimbursement attempted to avoid paying for the value associated with such status. Some of the flaws in these efforts will be discussed in the next section. Specifically, the capital reimbursement systems that emerged were based on actual audited costs, and a change of ownership did not affect that reimbursement.

Cost Control

New York City's financial crisis followed on the heels of the nursing home reform efforts. The state was forced to take stringent measures to protect its own solvency and to assure credit. Initially, nursing home rates were frozen in 1976 at 1975 levels. It was not until September 1976 that final rates for the year were promulgated. For the first time, voluntary and proprietary facilities were considered to be in the same cost categories. Stringent ceilings were imposed. Many voluntary homes and some proprietary homes were faced with retroactive reductions, rather than an increase over their 1975 rates. The objective of these efforts, although not explicitly stated, was to freeze gross expenditures for long-term care. That cost control objective was far more ambitious than were those imposed on any other part of the health sector.

Relating Reimbursement to Quality of Care

Creating a method of relating reimbursement to quality of care, as required by Chapter 649 of the 1975 nursing home reform laws, followed a chaotic course. (*McKinney's Session Law News of New York*, 1975) The development of a five-category rating system was originally intended for consumers' information. It was assumed by the Health Department that the linkage between quality of care and reimbursement would follow a different course. It was only during the spring of 1976, after the rating system had been almost completely developed, that there was a legislative mandate to tie it to reimbursement (*McKinney's Session Law News of New York* 1976, Chapter 76). The rating system was applied to reimbursement in 1976, 1977, and 1978. The method changed from year to year, with less difference in reimbursement between differently rated institutions each year.

Drafts of the proposed rating system were developed by a Health Department task force appointed by the commissioner and were reviewed in a series of meetings with the authors of the legislative bill, liaison committees of the major organizations of providers, and regional and county survey staffs. These preparations became diverted somewhat by the passage of Chapter 76, which specified that Title XVIII and XIX federal standards be used as the minimum standard and state hospital code be used as the maximum standard.

The so-called mini-maxi standard, a compromise in the efforts to control costs in 1976, required differentiation of the "good" rating into "good — federal" and "good — state." Ratings consisted of evaluation in eight areas: nursing, food-nutrition, leisure activities, cleanliness and safety, medical care, rehabilitation therapy, social work, and building features. Each of these areas was given one of five ratings ("very good", "good — state", "good — federal", "needs improvement", "unacceptable") in addition to an overall rating using the same five categories.

Reimbursement incentives differed in 1976, 1977, and 1978. They involved lower cost ceilings for those with lower ratings and higher ceilings for those with very good ratings.

At least on the surface, the intent had been carried out. The operators had been provided with a clear financial incentive to give higher quality care. The cumbersome appeal process and the delays necessary to impose fines on substandard operators had been circumvented. Operators would immediately feel the financial consequences of the quality of their operations.

Summary of Changes

Starting in 1976, a nursing home operator faced a strikingly different reimbursement environment. Independent civil and criminal investigations of financial transactions were being undertaken by a large, well-financed Special Prosecutor's office. Rather than a handful of Health Department auditors, the operators faced a combined Health Department and Office of the Special Prosecutor audit force of over 300 people. Capital costs were carefully scrutinized and limited to certified historical costs. Operators faced disallowances, based on audits, for costs in excess of what was judged to be prudent buying. Reimbursement rates would reflect the quality of care they provided. The overall rates no longer distinguished between types of ownership. Public expenditures were being held at 1975 levels. Finally, the nursing home investigations, the reorganizations of reimbursement, and the state's fiscal crisis had changed the climate in which operators and reimbursement regulators acted.

Results

A review of the impact of these diverse reforms will assess their effectiveness in controlling abuse, controlling costs, and linking quality of care to reimbursement.

Control of Abuse

It is difficult to assess impact of the 1975 laws aimed at controlling abuse. The requirement for full reporting of ownership in the annual financial reports may have discouraged some of the more blatant abuses. The prudent buyer concept in the evaluation of purchases proved difficult to put into operation and was abandoned when more stringent cost control legislation was passed the next year. The penalties for false financial statements and the liability of controlling persons no doubt encouraged greater caution in the completion of cost reports. The actual 1974 cost reports, submitted at the end of April 1975, revealed a discrepancy between reported costs and reimbursements of roughly $70 million (Hess, 23 May 1975, p.1). This was labeled "windfall profits" in the media, but it might be more appropriately described as "deterrent effect." Audit recoveries will be discussed in detail in the next chapter.

Efforts to control capital reimbursement abuses went through a series of refinements. The recommendations of the Public Health Council's ad hoc task force were adopted by the Health Department in March 1975 but were never fully implemented. The following are the basic tenets of their recommendations:

1. Medicaid capital cost reimbursement should be based on actual, certified costs.

2. Capital cost reimbursement to new facilities should consist of a rate of return on equity, depreciation, and reimbursement of actual interest on

authorized and approved financing. Reimbursement should be determined without regard to whether the facility is owned by the operator or leased and, if leased, without regard to the relationship between the owner and tenant.

3. The excess of reimbursement payments for depreciation over mortgage payments should be put in escrow and funded. This fund would provide money for the eventual replacement of the facility and for the payment of the mortgage when the proportion of the mortgage payments going to pay interest on the debt dropped and the proportion of those payments going towards amortization rose above the depreciation payments.

4. Once established for a facility, reimbursement rates should not change because of sale or lease. The funded depreciation requirement was imposed in order to assure that, since depreciation was based on a forty-year straight-line method at 2.5 percent per year, and since most mortgages have a twenty- to twenty-five-year term, funds would be available to pay the difference between amortization payment and allowable reimbursed depreciation. The proposal would have posed difficult administrative and legal problems in terms of sales, use as collateral, and administration of estates.

The Moreland Commission voiced a concern that the declining payments for capital costs might encourage some owners to convert perfectly acceptable nursing homes to other uses. Also, some kind of imputed rental system or way of paying an owner for the use of the facility would be required for older facilities without mortgages.

The Moreland Commission proposals, adopted in January 1976, attempted to deal with these problems. The so-called fair rental system was calculated by adding (i) 2.5 percent of allowed building and fixed equipment costs (forty-year depreciation of the costs), (ii) a rate of return on the unamortized costs equivalent to the Medicare rate of return (one and one-half times the average interest rates on federal securities held by the Federal Hospital Insurance Trust Fund), and (iii) a rate of return on land costs equivalent to the Medicare rate of return, adjusted for inflation.

While this method preserved the insulation of capital reimbursement from real estate transactions and lease arrangement and eliminated some of the incentives for early sale or conversion, it created other problems. First, it was not equitable. Older facilities that had lower interest mortgages or no mortgage at all benefited, while more recently constructed facilities with higher interest mortgages incurred losses. Banking interests and the New York Health Facilities Association, which represented most of the newly constructed proprietary homes, actively opposed the fair rental system. The joint executive and legislative task force on residential health care facilities was appointed by the governor to review the problems of the fair rental system in early 1977. Morton Hyman, the Public Health Council member whose ad hoc task force had produced the initial recommendations and who was a critic of the Moreland Commission recommendations, was named chairman. The senate, assembly, Health Department, and governor's office were represented on the task force. After extensive diagnostic and technical investigations, the task force produced a more flexible system that was used for calculating reimbursement in 1978.

Under this system, reimbursable capital costs for proprietary homes are determined by combining four factors: (i) interest on the capital indebtedness at a rate that the commissioner determines to be reasonable under the circumstance prevailing at the time of incurring that indebtedness, (ii) amortization of capital indebtedness, (iii) return on equity at a rate equal to the Medicare rate of return, and (iv) return of equity, given the characteristics and ability of the facility to meet its current capital indebtedness. The cumulative average annual payments for amortization and return of equity cannot, however, exceed 2.5 percent of the initial allowed capital cost of the facility.

The new regulations also give the Health Department flexibility in adjusting rates if they appear to produce excessive reimbursement or severe economic hardship. In the case of severe hardship, capital cost reimbursement may not exceed the debt service on allowable capital indebtedness. Provisions are also made for the estimation of fair and reasonable initial allowed capital cost for all facilities that are leased, where such cost data cannot be verified or are unavailable for other, acceptable reasons.

The evolution of these regulations illustrates the difficulty of dealing equitably with diverse, changing financial circumstances. The resulting synthesis appears to assure that the objectives of the reforms (elimination of trafficking, or rapid sale of homes as a form of real estate speculation, and sale to related parties to inflate one's capital cost reimbursement) are met without the initial inequities. The greater flexibility also implies a greater confidence in the ability of the Health Department to administer the program.

While the reforms have achieved their desired objectives, they have produced some unanticipated consequences. Whereas incentives for the rapid sale of homes have been eliminated, the Health Department now faces the reverse problem: it can't get rid of bad operators, even those who would clearly like to get out. Voluntary community groups have negotiated with the Health Department for purchase of some of these marginal operations. However, operators usually seek something comparable to current market value, and the Health Department will reimburse only historical cost. Few community groups can absorb this difference. The Health Department thus faces a dilemma: either continue to subsidize less than optimal care or, by altering capital reimbursement for voluntary community groups, assure a profit for the substandard and sometimes felonious operators. Health Department officials made an exception in the case of a facility that was purchased by a county and those officials faced an intensive investigation and possible prosecution by the Office of the Special Prosecutor, as will be described in Chapter Four. In another case, to be described in Chapter Five, a substandard nursing home was obtained by a community group by raising approximately $250,000 to make up the difference between the operator's price and the Health Department's reimbursement.

The tightening of capital reimbursement, however, has not resulted in wholesale conversions of nursing homes to other uses, as some have argued (Little 1975, p. 97). Some of the older wood frame facilities that were forced to close because of the Life Safety Code have been converted to other uses. Facilities built explicitly as nursing homes since the inception of the Medicaid program appear to be single-purpose buildings that are not easily convertible. Five of these more modern facilities that were closed, or were never allowed to open, remain empty. There was, however, widesperad removal of equity in the homes by owners in 1975. One operator removed over $1 million in equity in his home in the heat of the crisis. Some substandard operators, faced with Special Prosecutor and Health Department investigations, pursued this course even further, by bleeding the institution through not paying its bills while accumulating Medicaid payments. A somewhat analogous situation occurred in 1976 and 1977, when some voluntary nursing homes faced with serious problems related to the stringent reimbursement, stopped repaying their Article 28A loans to the state. The payment of those loans was built into the rate. A lock-box procedure was adopted by the state — continued reimbursement to the homes was made only under assurance of continued payment of the construction loans (Respondent 54 1978).

Thus, while there were efforts to cut or at least contain losses, there were few sales. Capital cost reimbursement constraints prevented operators from leaving the business. They have persisted, in hopes that favorable changes in reimbursement regulations will enable them to receive something closer to market value for their investments. The Health Facilities Association continues to press for movement in this direction, currently for the more beneficial component depreciation enjoyed by the voluntary nursing homes. Voluntary homes may depreciate certain capital costs over shorter intervals than the forty years imposed on all building costs for the proprietary nursing homes.

Control of Costs

As indicated in Figure 3.4, actual Medicaid expenditures by the state of New York for 1976 and 1977 dropped. These results are even more striking

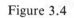

Figure 3.4

New York State Medicaid Payments from Fiscal Year
1966–67 to Fiscal Year 1978–79

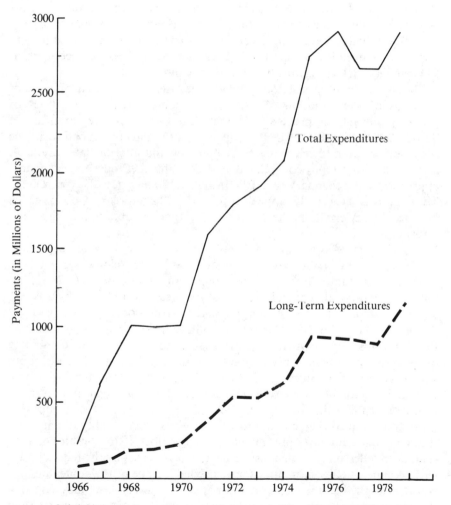

Included in long-term expenditures are skilled nursing facilities and intermediate care facilities.
Source: State of New York. Executive Budget. FY1965/6 to FY1978/9.

considering the average increase in expenditures in the program in earlier years.

The drop was not achieved without a price. Almost every health facility in the state filed rate appeals in 1976 and 1977. Article 78 procedures, by which a party may appeal a governmental administrative action in the courts, were implemented by the Hospital Association of New York, the New York Health Facilities Association, and the New York Association of Homes for the Aged. The New York Health Facilities Association brought a class action suit against the Commissioner of Health after the interim rates were frozen at 1976 and 1975 levels. The rates finally promulgated in September were even lower than the 1975 rates and required the recouping of $34.4 million in overpayments based on the interim rate.

The issues in the class action suit concerned the legality of changing rates in terms of the violation of contractual rights, depriving facilities of property without due process of law, and the violation of requirements in Section 249 (a) of P.L. 92–603, which require state participation in the Medicaid program to reimburse skilled nursing and intermediate care facilities on a "reasonable cost-related basis," using methods and standards approved by the secretary of HEW [*Kaye* v. *Whalen,* (1978, App. Div.)]. The suit was eventually appealed to the U.S. Supreme Court, which declined to review it in the fall of 1978, thereby upholding the state's position.

The Hospital Association of New York filed suit over similar issues involving the reasonable-cost aspects of New York's reimbursement. The association was initially successful in obtaining an additional $37 million, but it lost on appeal. The state's successful appeal was obtained by a Washington law firm for a cost of approximately $1 million.

The New York State Association of Homes for the Aged, whose members faced the most serious financial consequences as a result of the combining of proprietary, public, and voluntary institutions into a single cost group, was successful in getting some indirect relief from the courts. The federal class action suit requested a restraining order, claiming irreparable harm. In response to this suit, the Health Department reviewed the operations of those who claimed they could not continue to provide quality of care with the reimbursement rates promulgated in November 1976. An ad hoc process, later called management assessment, was required by the federal judge to determine whether more funds were needed for one of the homes and this was then applied by the Department of Health to the other homes named in the suit. Quarterly staffing reports, cost reports, inspection reports, and medical reviews were used in the assessments. The court instructed the Health Department to conduct similar assessments for the other homes in that class. The management assessment process became a permanent means of accommodating arguments of patient mix or other situations peculiar to facilities that were not accounted for in the rate-setting methodology. The process has been altered several times. Some homes, however, suffered major reductions that were not adjusted. The Division of the Budget study in 1978 criticized the process, since almost all assessment produced additional reimbursement for the facilities. There were some questions about the advisability of the program staff's being solely responsible for decisions concerning additional reimbursement. The Division of the Budget was concerned with plugging this potential source of leaks. A team approach using representatives from the central reimbursement group of the Health Department was being explored. For the first time, there was a direct link between cost control and quality assurance, functions that have operated in isolation from, and often at odds with, each other. The new process will either return to providers whatever has been taken away in terms of reimbursement controls; or give only lip service to issues of quality raised by tight reimbursement methods, while involving operators in fruitless maneuvering and containing increases in reimbursement; or balance these often conflicting goals.

In spite of the claims of imminent disaster, however, the industry appears to have survived. According to Health Department records, ten facilities have gone bankrupt between 1976 and 1979. Investigation of the details of each suggest that state fiscal controls were not the major cause for these failings. Three of the bankrupt facilities were connected through ownership to a national chain based outside of the state; the bankruptcy of the chain resulted in the bankruptcy of twenty facilities nationwide. Thus, conditions in New York State were not directly to blame for these three. Four of the bankrupt facilities involved operators who had been either indicted or convicted on charges related to Medicaid larceny or kickback schemes. Two involved an operator who had left the country and whom the state was unable to extradite to face charges of substandard care. There was a feeling on the part of Health Department officials that these homes may have been bled by the operator (that is, the operator may have pocketed portions of the Medicaid reimbursement rather than using it to pay operating expenses).

The remaining facility received a per diem rate in 1977 of $40.15; in spite of the facility's repeated appeals, the Health Department could find no justification for a rate increase. Rates for these bankrupt facilities in 1977 ranged from $27.14 for a health-related facility to $48.18 for the most costly skilled nursing facility; average reimbursement was over $38.00. All of the bankrupt homes were proprietary and were substantially larger than the average proprietary facility. The modal facility had over 200 beds, and the number of beds ranged from 80 to 520. Larger facilities generally have been assumed to be better able to deal with financial stringencies. Indeed, this was, according to some, part of the underlying rationale for the state Health Department's requiring a minimum of 60 beds for the licensure of new facilities.

Linking Reimbursement to Quality of Care

In the nursing home reform legislation signed into law in August 1975, there were requirements for the creation of a system of ratings intended for consumer information and a requirement that rates of reimbursement be tied to quality of care in the facilities. Development of the rating system by an ad hoc task force in the Health Department proceeded through the fall of 1975. Little attention was paid to the other requirement of the legislation because the Health Department felt that it was unrealistic. In early 1976, Commissioner of Health Robert Whalen indicated in a memorandum to the Assembly's Health Committee that it could not be done. This was not received well within the legislature. Reimbursement continued to operate separately from enforcement of standards. Had it not been for the fiscal crisis following so closely on the heels of the nursing home scandals, they might have continued to do so.

The governor's cost containment package in 1976 focused on the Medicaid program. Unlike social services or education, the Medicaid program had built-in adjustments for inflation. Thus, unless something was done, the cost of the program would go up, as it had been doing, at a rate of about 25 percent per year. The program amounted to 20 percent of the state budget. Private auditors were swarming through the Division of the Budget assessing the credibility of the state budget from the perspective of the banking industry (Respondent 49 1978). The need to demonstrate fiscal viability translated into the objective, unstated or cautiously expressed, of freezing the gross expenditures for the Medicaid program. Explicitly stated, this would not have been politically acceptable. Some maneuvering was required. The legislators did not want to lose the advances of the 1975 reforms. The package that emerged attempted to balance these forces.

First, attention was focused on reimbursement of providers rather than restriction of benefits or eligibility. Providers, it was felt, would be better able to absorb these cuts than would welfare recipients, and the nursing home exposés had made this alternative politically acceptable. Second, this constraint would be more palatable if there were some differential impact; that is, the good guys would be rewarded and the bad guys would be punished. The notion of a range of acceptable care emerged. The state would insist on a minimum standard and would be willing to pay up to a maximum standard. Initially, the federal standards would serve as the floor and the state standards would serve as the ceiling, but the commissioner was to initiate whatever changes were appropriate. The nursing home reimbursement issues of that legislation were the last to be resolved. The 1976 rates were finally filed as a part of the administrative rules and regulations on 30 September 1976 and were retroactive to 1 January 1976.

Facilities were grouped into five categories, based on number of beds, and costs were allocated to six functional areas: nursing, food-nutrition, leisure activities, cleanliness and safety, social work, and administration.

The ceilings on allowable costs depended on the quality ratings. Each facility's costs were compared to the per diem costs for the facilities in its size group that received a "good—state" rating. Table 3.1 shows the cost ceilings that were imposed.

Table 3.1

Cost Ceilings for Facilities, Based on Ratings.

Ratings	Percentile of appropriate group of facilities with good—state ratings
Unacceptable	10th
Needs improvement	25th
Good—federal	35th
Good—state	60th
Very good	No ceiling on allowable costs

Source: New York State Department of Health, Office of Health Systems Management, 1978d.

Ceilings imposed in prior years were relatively benign in comparison. Nursing service costs, the largest component, had been excluded from the cost component ceilings, and costs of other components were based on 110 percent of the average per diem component cost. Nursing service costs were, however, included in calculating the overall ceiling of 115 percent. Since the distribution of per diem costs is skewed to the right, the average per diem cost was somewhat above the 60th percentile. A 10 percent cushion on top of this made it a fairly mild constraint for most facilities. Adding to the shock was the grouping of voluntary, public, and proprietary homes together. In the past, they had been reimbursed separately. The voluntary and the proprietary homes had been regulated differently in terms of capital costs and standards, and allowable operating costs. Their costs reflected these differences. The public and voluntary institutions, whose per diems tended to be substantially higher than the proprietary institutions, now found themselves in the right tail of the per diem arrays for the new combined groupings. In many cases, the voluntary home rates for 1976, which were finally calculated in October 1976, were substantially below the frozen 1975 rates. The 1975 rates served as a basis for 1976 reimbursement in the interim, with the understanding that adjustments would be made when the final rates were calculated.

The impact of the rating system was substantially watered down in calculating reimbursement in 1978. The ratings were reduced to three categories and the differentials were also reduced. Overall ratings and overall ceilings were used instead of calculating on the basis of each functional area.

The distinctions between the mini-maxi notions, which were unaltered in the code, became difficult to justify and were eliminated. Thus, the notion of a range of acceptable care was watered down further. Since cost allocations in some of the categories were arbitrary, given the lack of uniform accounting, the overall ceilings and overall ratings were determined to be more accurate. The 1979 rates involved an inflation adjustment applied to the 1978 rates. The 1979 rates were less stringent for most homes. It was time for a breather, and the link between ratings and reimbursement rates became even more tenuous.

Operationally, the link between quality and reimbursement never received a fair test. There was substantial resistance to the idea at most levels in the Health Department. The link with the rating system was hastily put together and generated protest within the industry. The initial ratings by the surveyors had not been linked to reimbursement; they were linked after the fact. Animosity between operators and surveyors had grown since 1975 as a result of pressure on surveyors to bear down on the industry and the sometimes clumsy efforts of regional offices to show results. The rating materials still placed the major burden of judgments on the inspectors themselves. For example, in arriving at an overall evaluation of nursing, inspectors were expected to make ratings of fifteen elements of nursing care, each with a point value. The evaluator was then supposed to perform the following computations: "very good," double the assigned point value; "good," give the assigned point value; "needs improvement," subtract the assigned point value from the total score doubled; "unacceptable," subtract the assigned point value.

Overall ratings were then to be calculated on the basis of these total scores as follows: "very good," 180–232 (provided nothing is marked in the "needs improvement" category); "good," 100–179 (provided nothing is marked in "unaccaptable" category); "needs improvement," 58–99; "unacceptable," less than 58.

All items were linked to parts of the code. The first of the six major items in the nursing ratings was, for example:

1. The nursing care given provides for the patient's illnesses and for the restoration and protection of their physical and emotional well-being and is planned, administered, and provided nursing care in conformance with the stated general purposes and policies of the nursing home and with the physician's plans for the medical management of each patient [New York State Hospital Code 1976 Part 731.2(a)(1)(2)].

   Very good: There is evidence that the objectives of nursing care have been developed beyond the minimums and reflect attention to individualized patient care and have a sound restorative philosophy and are *implemented*.

   Good: There is evidence that these objectives are written and carried out as written.

   Needs improvement: There is evidence that the written objectives are not carried out or inconsistently carried out.

   Unacceptable: There are no objectives and no evidence that there is any goal for nursing care.

There was attached an explanation for surveyors of the discrepancy between compliance with federal standards ("good — federal") and compliance with state standards ("good — state"), so that such distinctions could be made in the ratings. In this particular case, there was essentially no difference between the relevant federal and state standards.

Similar ratings were carried out in seven other areas: food and nutrition, leisure time, cleanliness and safety, medical care, rehabilitation therapy, social work, and building features.

The flaws in the process are obvious and are acknowledged by all respondents: In spite of the lengthy, complex, time-consuming methodology, it is essentially subjective. Added to these problems were others. The rating task was added to the duties of the surveyors at a time when they were being drawn into many disputes with nursing homes concerning deficiencies, fines, and closing of facilities. No additional staff were added. The morale of the surveying teams was low. They felt put upon by the operators, harrassed by Albany, and placed in an impossible situation. Adaptation to these conditions varied among the six Health Department regional offices and the three county contract offices. In some, it ranged from conscientious, aggressive efforts to implement the rating system to passive sabotage, to even less veiled defiance, as described in Chapter Two.

The situation is comparable to one that might result from a university president's decreeing to students that tuition would be related to the grades they receive in their courses (those who received As would get free room and board and those who received Ds and Fs would have to pay double the normal cost) and grades would be based on essay exams evaluated by undergraduate graders.

Respondents who operate nursing homes viewed the rating process with disdain. It did not become a focus of hostility until it was linked to reimbursement.

The elaborate review and appeal process tended to mitigate against strict ratings by the surveyors. The ratings were first reviewed by a supervisor, then by the director of the long-term care program, and finally by the area administrator. Facilities were notified of their rating and had twenty days to appeal it to the area administrator. If not satisfied at this level of appeal, the facility could then appeal to the Commissioner of Health. The commissioner had appointed a rating appeal board composed of central staff in the program area. The facility was able to present to the board whatever evidence it felt was appropriate for review of its case. Appeal was almost automatic for facilities that received "need improvement" or "unacceptable" ratings. During the latter half of 1976, the rating appeal board was faced with almost sixty appeals. The appeals tapered off to about forty in 1977 and thirty in 1978. As in the other areas, there was a large backlog and many delays in the appeal reviews.

Problems with the rating system began to crop up, many of them predictable. There were stark differences in the distribution of the ratings. For example, as indicated in Table 3.2, seven out of nine facilities in the state with "very good" ratings in 1978 were in the White Plains region. It is hard

Table 3.2

Ratings for Skilled Nursing Facilities.

Rating	Region					
	Albany	Buffalo	Rochester	Syracuse	White Plains	New York City
Very good	1	0	0	0	7	1
Good — state	28	26	18	34	41	56
Good — federal	1	2	0	0	6	6
Needs improvement	0	0	0	0	1	6
Unacceptable	0	0	0	0	0	1
Deferred	2	0	0	0	1	0
Information not given	1	1	0	3	2	1

Source: New York State Department of Health, 1979.

to explain why the best facilities were concentrated in this region. Although ratings were supposed to be related to efficiency as well as quality, it was unclear how this was to be done; indeed, in some cases, it was doubtful that it was even attempted. Theoretically, it was conceivable to load up on nursing staff, get a "very good" rating and have all of these excessive costs reimbursed. This created a highly inflationary incentive within a legislative package that was supposed to contain costs. As soon as it became clear to the facilities and the inspectors that the ratings were used for reimbursement, the ratings began to converge. Not only were the incentives reduced in 1978, as compared to 1976 and 1977, but the number of facilities actually affected by the ratings, either positively or negatively, was reduced to a handful (see Table 3.3).

Table 3.3

Ratings for Skilled Nursing
and Health-related Facilities.

	Ratings												
	Very good		Good— state		Good— federal		Needs improvement		Un- acceptable		Other		Total*
Year	%	No.	%	No.	%	No.	%	No.	%	No.	%	No.	% No.
	Skilled nursing facilities												
1976	.4	2	59	324	28.2	155	6.2	34	3.3	18	2.9	16	100 549
1977	.7	4	79.7	432	13.5	73	4	20	1.8	10	.6	3	100 542
1978	3.4	17	88	446	7.1	36	4.5	23	1	5	.6	3	100 507
	Health-related facilites												
1976	.4	1	72.3	167	19	44	5.6	13	.4	1	2.2	5	100 231
1977	.9	2	83.9	193	10.9	24	3.5	8	0	0	.9	2	100 230
1978	3.8	9	84.7	200	6.8	16	3	7	.4	1	1.3	3	100 236

* Total may not equal 100% because numbers are rounded off.
Source: New York State Department of Health, 1979.

Overall, ratings tended to rise. Health Department and industry spokespersons found themselves in the somewhat contradictory position of using these trends to argue that the abuses of the past had been corrected, while at the same time arguing that the harsh reimbursement system imposed on the industry in 1976 had threatened the system with deterioration in quality. None of the respondents interviewed within the department or the industry expressed much faith in the reliability of ratings. Nor did any feel that the ratings provided an effective financial incentive for delivering high quality care. There was disagreement among respondents, however, about whether the system had really been given a fair trial.

The system did, however, help bring into focus the issues surrounding attempts to link reimbursement to quality of care.

Respondents conceded the power of reimbursement incentives on providers. There is no problem in getting complete, timely fiscal reports; if an operator does not complete the reports, he will not be reimbursed. Compliance with these requirements far outshadows compliance with any of the quality of care standards imposed by the Health Department code. Fines can be appealed, and the Health Department has not been particularly successful in making them stick. It has been even more time-consuming and difficult to close noncomplying facilities.

Why not simply force substandard facilities to shut down by cutting off reimbursement? The impact would be immediate. The facilities could appeal, but in this case the lengthy and cumbersome appeal process would work against them. The operators would either respond to these reimbursement incentives and upgrade their facilities, or go bankrupt. The facilities would be forced to close without going through the efforts of removing licenses. Why shouldn't the state use the most powerful weapon it has at its disposal?

Such an approach, however, ignores the rationale for standards and reimbursement. The Health Department's function in policing the facilities is to protect the welfare of the patients and to assure that those who cannot care for themselves are properly cared for. Cutbacks in the reimbursements to substandard facilities could result in cutbacks in nurse staffing and food budgets rather than in the profits of operators. In the last analysis, the patients are the hostages of the substandard operator. It was this concern for the nursing home residents that subverted the rating system, once rating was tied to reimbursement, and that contributed to the ambivalence of the Health Department as a whole in implementing the program. Legislation passed in 1980 at the request of the Office of Health Systems Management substituted a more qualitative consumer information system for the rating system proposed by the 1975 legislation.

Conclusions

The previous sections have reviewed the problems faced by the reimbursement system for nursing homes in New York, the methods that were developed to deal with those problems, and the results of the implementation or attempted implementation of the proposed solutions. This section will review more informally the general issues and lessons in that process.

Many of the errors appear to be inherent in large bureaucratic organizations, where problems are factored into manageable pieces, and where the search for solutions is limited and focused on standard operating procedures. Thus, the Division of the Budget's limited focus resulted in rejection of the requested audit positions in the early 1970s. The management assessment process — indeed, the entire standards-setting process — suffered from its isolation from fiscal issues. Efforts such as the interdisciplinary teams for management assessment, brought about in part by external pressures, are an attempt to deal with the dysfunction resulting from such fragmentation.

The reimbursement and quality of care dilemma suggests an analogy. Three individuals are stranded on a desert island without water or food. A raft floats ashore carrying cans of food and water. Opening the containers presents a problem. The first two individuals suggest either throwing the water cans up in the air so that they will smash open or smashing them with rocks: Neither course would be successful, since most likely the water would be lost. The third individual has a Ph.D. in economics, and the others turn to him for advice. After a thoughtful pause, he replied, "Assume that you have a can opener."

Assume that you have a method for accurately and consistently measuring the quality of care and for decreasing reimbursement to substandard facilities in such a way so that only the controlling persons would be affected. Is it possible? We are now limited to indirect ways of measuring quality, like measuring a flickering shadow, while its essence eludes us. The more we attempt to measure it objectively (that is, width of corridors, fire resistance ratings of building materials, professional degrees earned by staff), the less confident we feel. Measures of outcome, rather than structural or process criteria, are supposed to be the solution. If bad outcomes for patients are avoided and good ones obtained, then we know that high quality care, whatever that is, has been provided. But have we really escaped from the measurement trap? Certainly, the movement of patients along a continuum from dependence to independence is encouraging, but does that represent quality? We can count and weigh such attributes. We can, with considerably more difficulty, combine them into a single number or measure. Will we feel sufficiently comfortable with that number to use the power of reimbursement for achieving it? Can something that is subjective and as ephemeral as quality really be measured at all? The main character in the novel *Zen and the Art of Motorcycle Maintenance* was driven crazy by that basic dilemma (Pirsig 1974). Those who pursue the goal of objective measurement of the quality of nursing home care may well meet the same fate.

Assume that the first goal is achieved, or at least satisfactorily approximated. Can we assure that financial penalties will not be borne by the

patients? We could, for example, reduce the salaries or return on investments that could be allocated to controlling persons. At least in dollar
terms, that might assure that the reductions would not be taken out of
patient care. But what about the indirect effects? Will loss of salary and
return on investment produce the added effort that is necessary to improve
care, or will it produce a reduced effort on the part of those controlling
persons? The answer is not clear-cut. Some marginal operators faced with
fines in 1976 and 1977 chose to bleed the institution (that is, stop paying
bills, obtain second mortgages at higher than reimbursable levels, and accu-
mulate reimbursement payments) and walk away. If an operator does not
bleed the institution of financial resources, he might still choose to bleed it
by reducing his effort. Even with both of these conditions crudely met, a
conscientious regulator, concerned about the patients in that home, might
well think twice before turning in a low rating.

No issue is as laden with emotion or as hotly debated as the role of proprietary homes. Some of the initial legislative recommendations in 1975
suggested phasing out the proprietary sector completely. This plan was
dropped when it became clear that it was not financially feasible.

The evidence in favor of or against profit-making operations, both in
terms of cost and quality, is somewhat ambiguous. Fifty-four percent of the
facilities in the state are proprietary. All eighteen of the long-term care facilities in receivership as of May 1979 for financial or quality of care
deficiencies are proprietary. The continuing violation hearings involved
eight proprietary and one voluntary facility. On the other hand, seven of the
nine facilities in the state receiving the highest ratings by the Health
Department in December 1978 were proprietary; the other two were voluntary. The only facility receiving the lowest rating, "unacceptable," during
this period was a proprietary institution. Besides this easily contested evidence, the most knowledgeable individuals interviewed give the impression
that proprietary facilities, in terms of quality of care, include some of the
very best and some of the very worst in the state.

The Moreland Commission conducted an elaborate analysis of the comparative costs by ownership in 1974 (see Table 3.4). A regression analysis
suggested, however, that most of these cost differences could be explained
by the different sizes of the structures and their geographic location
(Moreland Act Commission 1976c, p. 43). After the Medicaid program was
begun, proprietary facilities faced tighter controls in terms of capital costs.
Reimbursement rates for voluntary and public facilities included costs for
medical directors, full time house staffs in many cases, and other expenses
not allowed proprietary facilities. Since the elimination of groupings by
ownership in 1976, the discrepancy between proprietary and voluntary
public rates has tended to narrow. It would seem that, if proprietary facil-

Table 3.4

Comparative Costs per diem of Skilled Nursing and
Health-related Facilities, by Ownership, 1974.

Ownership	Facility	
	Skilled nursing ($)	Health-related ($)
Voluntary	44.93	20.28
Proprietary	29.57	18.90
Public	39.32	24.15

Source: Moreland Act Commission, 1976c, pp. 42, 64.

ities were more efficient producers of services, the rate-setting system, rather than the alleged natural superiority of the profit sector, made them so. Even though attention was initially focused on fraud in the proprietary sector, investigations by the Office of the Special Prosecutor in the Willow Point case discussed in Chapter Four, suggest that fraud need not be unique to the for-profit sector.

Finally, although voluntary homes argued for higher reimbursement rates than those of proprietary facilities because of more seriously ill and, consequently, more costly patients, data collected in Health Department surveys of patient characteristics do not support this argument (Respondent 69 1978).

In retrospect, there is something appealing about local social service commissioners negotiating with area homes for the care of welfare patients at a fixed charge, based largely on what they felt they could afford. Some of the operators whose names were closely linked with substandard care and Medicaid fraud reportedly never felt comfortable with the cost-based system (Respondent 47 1979). They preferred the old fixed-charge patterns. There appears to be a retreat from cost-based reimbursement for long-term care. Neither system avoids the need for control. Cost-based reimbursement without proper auditing invites fraud. Charge-based reimbursement without adequate monitoring of quality invites substandard care. In a negotiated rate system, the patients become the victims. Substandard care was the issue, for example, in the Kaplan investigations in New York City in the late 1950s. By contrast, the 1974 scandals involved primarily financial dealings. The state should be better able to defend itself against fraudulent cost-reporting and inflated capital costs than against substandard care. The more one squeezes reimbursement, the more attention must be paid to quality. As with public utility regulation, little emphasis has been placed on regulating the quality of the product. It is assumed, in most cases, a firm has a financial incentive to improve quality (Kahn 1971, pp. 1, 21, 25): so it is with cost-related reimbursement of health care. Whether those increases in cost and quality are affordable is another question.

Health care reimbursement has become a new form of warfare. Accountants and lawyers have become the mercenaries. Whoever has the most resources, the most skilled mercenaries, wins. The Health Department, by hiring a law firm for over $1 million, was able to prevent the hospitals in New York from recapturing approximately $30 million in funding. The stakes are high, and the Health Department, like any other public regulatory agency, is at a disadvantage. It has become the training ground for the industry. One former Health Department accountant has become the president of a small chain, and the Health Department's counsel has become a partner in the law firm that represented several key operators who were convicted of fraud and bribery. There has been a substantial turnover of key people in the rate-setting section, as many have gone to work for providers. One auditor, who had disallowed certain expenditures for a home, has now been hired by the home to handle the appeal of those findings. Civil service salaries cannot compete with others in the industry. People who have had experience on the inside are extremely valuable to people outside. The situation is hardly unique to New York. In Missouri, for example, the former chairman of the state board of health (responsible for licensing nursing homes) formed a nursing home management firm and then hired the director of health planning and the individual responsible for developing the state's Medicaid cost-related nursing home reimbursement plan. The firm also hired a nursing home inspector and a nursing home auditor from the same state agency (Ganey 1978).

Finally, it helps to know where you are going. Efforts to freeze gross expenditures were effective because they started with that objective and then massaged the reimbursement system to achieve it. As indicated in Figure 3.5, there is a cyclical pattern in efforts to control Medicaid expenditures that perhaps reflects broader political realities. Growth in Medicaid expenditures, particularly in terms of expenditures for nursing homes, have followed a four-year cycle since the inception of the program (Figure 3.5). Increases peak in the year of a gubernatorial election and dip in a mid-term election year. Labor union settlements and the need for labor support were suggested by several respondents as a factor in this cycle. As the four-year moving average suggests, however, there has been a dampening effect on increases since the inception of the program. While the cyclical political influence on expenditures in the program remains, it appears to be increasingly restrained by cost controls.

Figure 3.5

New York State Medicaid Payments for Nursing Home Care
from Fiscal Year 1966–67 to Fiscal Year 1978–79,
by Percent Increase

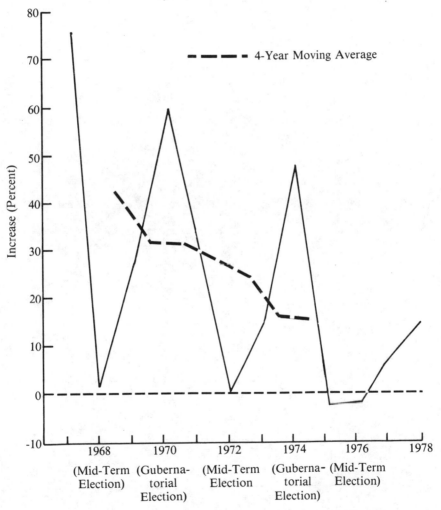

Included are Skilled Nursing Facilities (SNF) and Intermediate Care Facilities (ICF).

Reimbursement controls and incentives clearly have limited influence on the performance of providers. The next chapter will deal with more coercive alternatives.

Chapter Four

Strengthening Criminal Enforcement

The relationship between New York State and the nursing home industry, from the state's point of view, was not unlike that between a permissive parent and a spoiled child. The parent patiently explains how he expects the child to behave. The parent may offer to give the child an extra allowance for being polite and helpful to company. If neither persuasion nor the extra dollars work, the parent may, in anger, beat the child.

In 1974 a similar sort of frustration led New York State to create the Office of the Special Prosecutor. The professional controls described in Chapter Two had proven relatively ineffective. Financial rewards did not appear to be particularly effective alternatives, as shown in Chapter Three. The only recourse seemed to be coercion, the threat of punishment: "Nail the bad apples and scare the hell out of the rest." Just as the actions of an enraged parent can have unintended consequences, so did the efforts to strengthen criminal enforcement described in this chapter. A national effort, modeled after New York's Office of the Special Prosecutor, was initiated in 1978. These changes were the most profound in the regulatory environment not only of nursing homes, but of the entire health sector.

Background

The history of prosecution in the nursing home sector before 1974 was a history of dust-collecting recommendations. In 1958 the New York City Commissioner of Investigations, Louis I. Kaplan, began a two-year probe of the proprietary nursing homes in the city. On 6 April 1960, Kaplan submitted his report to Mayor Robert F. Wagner. It was a damning indictment of the proprietary nursing home industry and the small group of operators who appeared to control it. The report made the following observations, as highlighted by the Temporary State Commission on Living Costs and the Economy some fifteen years later (1975, pp. 132–34):

1. Many operators were attracted purely by the opportunity to make substantial returns on capital investments and were neither socially motivated nor professionally equipped for the undertaking.

2. Public regulation, because of the profit incentive, had to become more vigorous if the public interest was to be served.

3. Proprietary nursing homes were inadequately staffed and were not qualified to carry out their responsiblities; the Department of Welfare and the Department of Hospitals had not assured the well-being of patients by enforcing code requirements.

4. Nursing homes filed attendance records that had been deliberately falsified to assure licensure from the Department of Hospitals and appropriate classification for referrals from the Department of Welfare.

5. Nursing homes failed to give patients the care they contracted with the Department of Welfare to provide and thus overcharged the department and the city of New York.

6. Proprietary nursing homes were controlled by a cartel of promoters concerned only with profit.

7. Twenty-five homes were controlled by one owner who never held a license in any of his homes and whose financial investments were recorded in the names of friends and relatives.

8. Nursing home operators had committed crimes by filing false reports and false instruments. Many freely admitted to Kaplan's investigators that they had committed such crimes. "Just about everyone admitted to filing false documents," said one of the investigators.

9. Between 1 July 1956 and 30 June 1958, these operators fraudulently overcharged the city $3.7 million. Kaplan recommended that (i) the city take steps to collect these overcharges and not increase payment to operators until the money had been recouped and that (ii) the report be forwarded to the New York County District Attorney's office so that criminal prosecution could be initiated.

The report was filed but never reached the attention of the District Attorney. While no prosecution resulted from the investigation, other steps were taken, including revision of the nursing home code (later to be used as a model for the state code), an increase in the number of inspectors, the closing of some substandard homes, improvement of in-service education and training programs for nursing home employees, and reorganization of city departments involved in regulation.

In 1962 the Department of Investigations conducted a follow-up to Kaplan's investigation. It reported no improvement in the operations of nursing homes. Rates had been increased to $265 per month, and the city had not recouped any of the alleged fraudulently obtained reimbursement. By 1964, only $626,878 of approximately $3.7 million in fraudulent overcharges had been recovered, and two rate increases had taken place. "We did the best we could," said Jan Abberman, one of the principal investigators, ". . . but we failed" (Temporary State Commission on Living Costs and the Economy 1975, p. 139).

The passage of Article 28 in New York State, as well as the enactment of Medicare and Medicaid in 1965, caused a basic shift in efforts to police the nursing home industry. Control shifted from the municipal and county health and welfare departments to the state Health Department. A statewide cost-related reimbursement system was established in 1966. At the same time, the state Health Department assumed primary responsibility for the standard of care within the facilities. The transition produced a temporary truce between regulators and the industry. Between 1966 and 1969, staff were added to the Health Department to perform the standards surveillance and rate-setting functions. The industry began to learn how to work within the new structure. It was a period of mutual adaptation.

The initial objectives of the state's regulatory efforts were to phase out facilities that did not meet basic life safety standards and to develop a complement of physical plants that would fully comply with federal and state standards.

Between 1967 and 1971, the Health Department was unable to conduct field audits. Desk reviews performed by rate-setting staff were relied upon to control abuse. The Bureau of Audits and Investigations was established in 1971 with a staff of eight. Audits in 1973 of a small number of homes uncovered significant overpayments. One of these initial audits, for example, revealed over $1 million in overstated costs that had allegedly been used to pay, among other things, an operator's alimony and fuel bills for a yacht in Florida. This was referred to the Attorney General for criminal prosecution, but no action was taken (Respondent 73 1979).

Concern with possible criminal prosecution did not surface again until 1974. In part, this was the result of the Temporary State Commission on Living Costs and the Economy, which had been created by the legislature and Governor Rockefeller in 1973 and which focused its investigations on nursing homes. During the summer and fall of 1974, investigations shifted from substandard care and the need for a nursing home ombudsman program to financial fraud, particularly fraudulent real estate transactions. These concerns were an outgrowth of investigations that had first been conducted by the establishment committee of the Public Health Council and later by an ad hoc committee to review capital cost financing. A particularly flagrant example of inflated construction costs of nursing homes came to the attention of the group. About $2.5 million of what was alleged to be "water" was squeezed out of the initially reported construction cost of $6 million (Respondent 45 1978).

During this same period a *New York Times* reporter, John Hess, was doing his own research. After contacting a Health Department official for permission to go through its records and talk to its staff, he was given free rein, but the official added, in frustration, "I don't really think anybody cares" (Respondent 73 1979).

On 10 September 1974, Hess published the first in a series of articles concerning nursing homes in the state. It was the beginning of an avalanche of press coverage of nursing homes. This wave of exposés differed substantially from previous ones in that it focused less on the plight of the residents than on the money flowing into the system and the role of politicians in protecting operators against vigorous enforcement. Hess paid particular attention to the opportunities for fraud and financial abuse by operators.

Jack Newfield, writing for the *Village Voice,* was less circumspect in his approach to what he perceived as corruption of public officials. He focused his attack on Attorney General Louis Lefkowitz and on Speaker of the Assembly Stanley Steingut, as well as on operators such as Bernard Bergman, Eugene Hollander, and Charles Sigety. "The current investigations into nursing homes should not concentrate exclusively on Bernard Bergman's empire. It is the whole ghoulish, politically protected industry that is corrupt, and it needs to be purified by a prosecutor who has a passion for justice" (Newfield 13 January 1975, p. 14). Newfield praised the selection of Charles Hynes for the job and described him as a "perfect prosecutor."

As suggested in Figures 4.1 and 4.2, press attention hit the nursing home industry like a tidal wave toward the end of 1974 and was sustained through 1976. The disproportionate share of this attention was focused on alleged criminal activity by public officials and operators. In contrast, the Kaplan investigation had caused scarcely a ripple in the press.

For the first time since the Kaplan investigations, the nursing home industry began to face sustained political pressure. It was a gubernatorial election year. The summer of 1974 was the culmination of the Watergate investigations. Richard Nixon was finally forced to resign as President in August 1974. Investigative reporters were the new cultural heroes; special prosecutors were seen as a vehicle for change. Paranoia concerning public officials and the programs they oversaw was at a peak.

Corruption in the Medicaid program and in the nursing home industry became one of the key issues of the election year. Several legislative candidates held news conferences on the steps of the Towers Nursing Home, a

Figure 4.1

New York Times Articles Dealing with Criminal Aspects
of the Nursing Home Situation in New York State, 1956–78

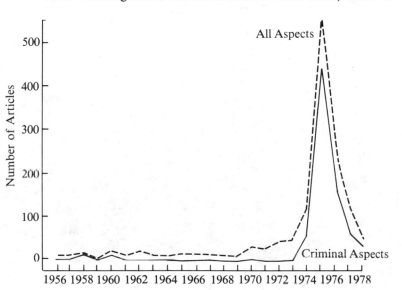

"Criminal aspects" include investigations, prosecutions, allegations of influence, and legislative
and court activities dealing with fraud and abuse, corruption, and political influence.

Bergman facility, labeling it a fire trap and attacking the laxity in the
enforcement of standards (*New York Times* 22 August 1974, p. 15). "Doing
something" about the nursing home issue became a campaign promise of
Democratic gubernatorial candidate Hugh Carey. Nursing home abuse
served as a convenient, concrete focus for the public's more amorphous
post-Watergate outrage.

Governor-elect Carey requested that Mario Cuomo, the designated secretary of state, prepare a report on the nursing home industry. Cuomo's
report echoed most of the newspaper charges of financial abuse and political impropriety. Cuomo alluded to nursing home syndicates as puppeteers
pulling political strings. "Who the mysterious overrulers are remains officially undisclosed, but there is no doubt of the existence of conflict of interest
ties involving officials of both parties" (Prial, 17 January 1975, p. 30).
Three specific recommendations from Cuomo's report, the creation of a

Figure 4.2

Percent of *New York Times* Articles that Deal with Criminal Aspects
of the Nursing Home Situation in New York State, 1956–78

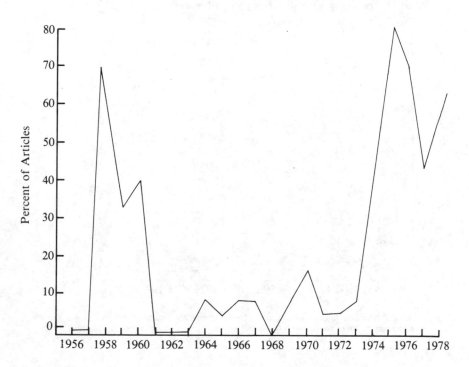

Moreland Act Commission to examine the nursing home and Medicaid
system, the appointment of a special prosecutor to investigate possible criminal charges, and the hiring of additional auditors for the Health Department, were adopted immediately.

On 10 January 1975, the first action of the new governor was the appointment of a special prosecutor. Charles Hynes, who had worked on rackets
investigations in Kings County was appointed Deputy Attorney General of
the State of New York, to act as special prosecutor under the authority of
Section 63 (3) of executive law. A new phase in the regulation of health care
providers began.

Originally, the Office of the Special Prosecutor (OSP) was given powers
to investigate nursing homes and vendors to the industry and had the unique
executive power to subpoena individuals and relevant books and records.
This was later upheld by the courts.

By the end of the first year, the staff of the OSP had grown to 208, including 64 auditors and 36 attorneys (Hynes 1976, p. 5). The staff had been organized into seven regional offices (New York City, Hauppague, Pearl River, Albany, Syracuse, Rochester, and Buffalo).

The structure of the OSP is indicated in Figure 4.3. The organizational chart gives a somewhat distorted picture, however, since the working structure is far more informal, with more open lines of communication than those suggested by the chart. (Indeed, no formal organizational chart existed before this one was drawn.) Special assistant attorneys general head the regional offices, which are staffed by additional lawyers, as well as investigators and auditors. The special assistant attorneys general were accountable to Hynes. The investigators and auditors also worked under the guidance, policy, and procedures developed at the state level by the executive staff. Investigators were recruited from the Federal Bureau of Investigation and from detective divisions of municipal police departments. The smallness of the regional staff and the emphasis on a team approach to cases appear to have alleviated some of the problems of coordination. Investigators, lawyers, and auditors worked together on cases at all stages, assuring a more coordinated approach than would normally take place in a district attorney's office.

Invitations to operators and others connected with nursing homes for informal conversation were usually ignored. In most cases, office subpoenas had to be issued. Subpoenas of financial records proved particularly torturous. Legal action by operators to quash subpoenas delayed investigations. In one case, this legal maneuvering consumed more than three years and resulted in the apparent disappearance of some of these records (Hynes 1977, p. 31).

The role of the OSP expanded significantly in 1976. On 12 April 1976, the legislature passed the special enabling legislation requested by Governor Carey to permit the hiring of an additional 146 staff to assist in the audit of proprietary nursing home cost claims submitted between 1969 and 1975. In June 1976, investigations were expanded to include private proprietary homes for adults, as well as nursing facilities.

The activities of the OSP quickly attracted federal attention. Section 17 of the Medicare-Medicaid Fraud and Abuse Bill of 1977 uses it as a model for developing legislation to encourage other states to create long-term fraud control units. According to the House Committee on Interstate and Foreign Commerce, "The Committee was particularly impressed with the organization and operation of the New York Special Prosecutor's Office, and believes it constitutes a model for anti-fraud efforts in other states" (U.S., Congress, House of Representatives 1977, p. 80). Section 17 provided for 90 percent federal funding of state anti-fraud programs similar to

Figure 4.3

Organizational Chart of the Office of the Special Prosecutor

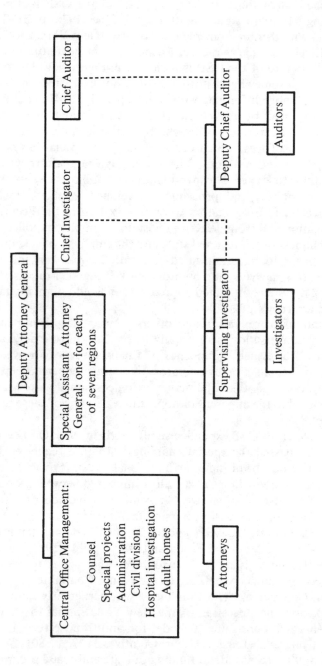

the OSP over a three-year period. The OSP became certified as the fraud control unit in New York State on 3 August 1978. As a result, its responsibilities were expanded beyond nursing homes, hospitals, and private proprietary homes for adults to include physicians, clinical laboratories, pharmacies, and other Medicaid providers who had previously been outside their jurisdiction. By the end of 1979, twenty-six other states had established fraud control units essentially modeled after New York's OSP. The OSP has been involved extensively in training and consulting with these new agencies.

The OSP nursing home investigations, which began in January 1975, focused on three areas: fraudulent use of Medicaid funds, patient abuse, and inappropriate intervention of public officials on behalf of nursing home operators.

For the first time, nursing homes faced a well-financed and well-organized group whose role was neither to consult nor to encourage efficient production of services, but to conduct investigations with the possibility of criminal prosecution. For the first time, the operator was not perceived as a professional colleague in need of assistance, or as an economic decision-maker, but as a possible criminal.

As summarized in Tables 4.1 and 4.2, the staff and budget of the OSP grew dramatically. Its designation as the Medicaid fraud control unit for New York State completed its evolution from a temporary investigative body to an apparently permanent fixture with which nursing homes and other Medicaid-eligible providers must come to terms.

Convictions

As of January 1980 the OSP had obtained indictments of 209 individuals for Medicaid fraud and related crimes (Respondent 75 1980). In the 155 completed cases, there have been 135 convictions, 11 acquittals and 9 dismissals (Respondent 75 1980). Of these indictments, 117 were related to nursing homes. These nursing home indictments involved 136 defendants and 102 nursing homes. These cases have resulted in 94 convictions, 7 dismissals, and 6 acquittals. Twenty cases are still pending. The prosecutions involved what the OSP described as "a predominantly three-pronged system to defraud Medicaid, involving personal luxury, fraud, kickbacks and pyramiding" (Hynes 1979, p. 11).

The largest proportion of indictments dealt with personal luxury fraud. For example, one operator, according to the OSP, billed more than $250,000 in personal expenditures to Medicaid. These expenditures included the purchase of a wedding cake, bridal gown, and flowers for his daughter,

Table 4.1

Budgets for the Office of the Special Prosecutor.

Fiscal year (April 1–March 31)	State funds ($1,000,000s)	Explanation for major budget shifts
1975–76	3.6	Initial budget
1976–77	6.2	Jurisdiction expanded to include audit of proprietary nursing home sector and private proprietary homes for adults. (June 28, 1976)
1977–78	7.1	Establishment of Civil Recovery Division (September 1, 1977)
1978–79	7.7	Patient abuse investigations expanded as a result of new reporting law (March 1978)
		Designated Medicaid fraud control unit for New York State. Responsibilities expanded to include all Medicaid providers (August 3, 1978)
1979–80	8.6	
1980–81	8.6 (proposed)	Completion of proprietary nursing home audits and recoveries, resulting in some reductions in staff

Figures include federal cost-sharing, which increased to 90 percent in 1978, but exclude fringe benefits, which run approximately 20 percent of salaries. Also excluded is the Health Care Financing Administration contract to investigate hospitals, which added $1.5 million in 1977–78, $3.0 million in 1978–79, $2.5 million in 1979–80, and $.5 million in 1980–81.

Source: New York State Department of Health, Office of the Special Prosecutor 1980.

veterinary bills for his horses, dog kennel bills, and shoeing expenses for his horses (Hynes 1978a, p. 14). The operator arranged to have the firms supplying these services bill one of his facilities, altering the bill so as to make it appear that they were legitimate facility expenses. Such expenditures, professionally doctored, are difficult for auditors to catch.

The most bizarre and most publicized case came to light when the curiosity of auditors was aroused by invoices that identified 100 lithographs costing an average of $150 each. The operator informed the auditors that these had been purchased to brighten up the environment for residents in his homes. Health Department inspectors, however, reported that they had seen nothing resembling lithographs in these four homes, only a few inexpensive cardboard scenes hung in various locations. The vendor, located in the the wealthy gallery district of New York City, was at first uncooperative, but he finally admitted that he had sold paintings, including a Renoir,

Table 4.2

Staffing Levels in the
Office of the Special Prosecutor
at the Beginning of the Calendar Year.

Staff	Year				
	1976	1977	1978	1979	1980
Attorneys	36	59	–	–	–
Special investigators	47	94	–	–	–
Special auditor-investigators	64	147	–	–	–
Management, administrative, and support	60	117			
Total	207	417	422	423	412*

*To be reduced to 376 by June 1980.

Source: Hynes 1976, 1977; New York State Department of Health, Office of the Special Prosecutor 1980.

to the operator and had made the invoices out for many cheaper lithographs addressed to the nursing home (Hynes 1979, p. 13). An additional Renoir, an Utrillo, and a Cassatt had found their way into the operator's collection through similar arrangements.

Other items, such as food for an operator's family, transportation (that is, yachts and Mercedes Benz automobiles), trips unrelated to business (vacations in the Bahamas), and educational expenses unrelated to the provision of patient care (an operator's son's college tuition), found their way, in doctored form, into the Medicaid cost reports of some facilities.

The use of Medicaid funds, designed to provide help for the medically indigent, to support the luxurious life-styles of operators makes for shocking headlines and emotional rhetoric. As in most areas where public funds are used, there is a continuum, ranging from rigid compliance with the letter of the law (which, because of changing regulations and interpretations, was, according to most respondents who were operators, impossible), to pristine compliance with at least the spirit of the law, to sloppy bookkeeping practices (particularly in the smaller, less tightly managed homes), to self-serving misinterpretation, to questionable ethical practices, to clearly premeditated fraud, and, finally, to uncontrolled looting. Where the majority of the operators fell along this continuum is a matter of sharp disagreement among respondents, but clearly the lack of effective audit controls, which was well understood by those in the industry, encouraged a drift toward the latter end of the continuum.

As of 10 May 1979, investigations into kickbacks have resulted in indict-

ments of fifty-two individuals and convictions of forty-one. Figure 4.4
shows how the kickback system works. The tactics adopted were similar to
those later used by the Federal Bureau of Investigation in its ABSCAM
investigations of political corruption.

A nursing home administrator facing sentencing for other criminal
charges cooperated as an undercover agent in the investigation. Fifty nursing home suppliers were targeted for contact by the agent. These fifty were
selected from a list of those suppliers who restricted their businesses to nursing homes and from a list of firms whose ownership was questionable. The
undercover agent then contacted the vendors, indicating that he was constructing a new nursing home and would like to know what kind of special
deals they could provide. Most of the vendors were all too willing to discuss
the special arrangements that could be made. The conversations were taped
and led to the indictment and conviction of thirty vendors, with no acquittals to date (Respondent 75 1980). The candor and openness of the suppliers
was surprising, given the intensive attention that had been focused on
nursing homes. Prosecutions exposed kickbacks ranging from $400 over
two months to $335,000 over six years (Hynes 1979, p. 16).

Kickback arrangements with suppliers followed one of three avenues.
First, arrangements could be made for inflated billings, in which cases
invoices exceeded the actual price of the goods purchased. The operator
could then receive a cash kickback and proceed to submit the inflated bills
in his Medicaid cost reports. Second, arrangements could be made with a
supplier for phony billings; that is, the operator could pay bills for nonexistent goods or services and then receive an under-the-table cash kickback.
Finally, phony items could be submitted along with regular invoices, with
the same method of sharing the spoils. Receipt of an unlawful kickback
remains a misdemeanor, with punishment limited to one year in jail, in spite
of efforts by the OSP to get legislation to increase the penalty.

Relatively few of the OSP's convictions have involved schemes to inflate
real estate or construction costs to the advantage of the owner or
non-arm's-length parties. Eight such convictions have been obtained in
nursing home schemes, resulting in excessive capital cost reimbursement of
between $1 and $2 million (Respondent 75 1980). In several cases the
caution of the Health Department in not relying completely upon the financial reports of facilities has worked against the OSP in obtaining convictions or recoveries based on misinformation in these reports. It has also
proved extremely difficult to explain to a grand jury the system used at a
particular time because of the complexity and constantly changing nature of
the systems. In several cases, all parties were thoroughly confused by the
end of grand jury testimony (Respondent 45 1980).

Figure 4.4

The Medicaid Kickback Scheme

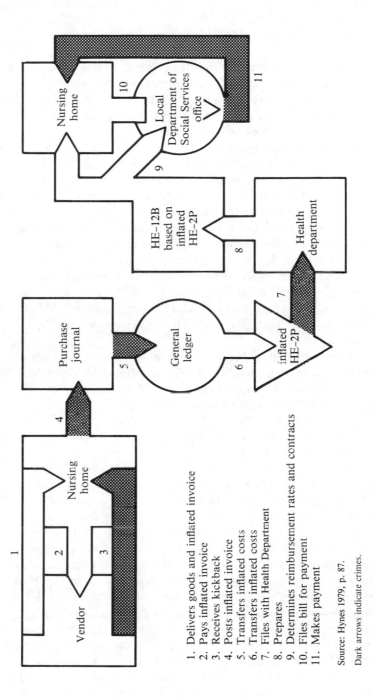

1. Delivers goods and inflated invoice
2. Pays inflated invoice
3. Receives kickback
4. Posts inflated invoice
5. Transfers inflated costs
6. Transfers inflated costs
7. Files with Health Department
8. Prepares
9. Determines reimbursement rates and contracts
10. Files bill for payment
11. Makes payment

Source: Hynes 1979, p. 87.

Dark arrows indicate crimes.

Recouping Fraudulent Medicaid Payments

Since there is a five-year statute of limitations on initiation of reimbursement-related prosecution for larceny or related felonies, the investigations had to focus on cost claims made in the financial reports of 1969 to 1975. Three hundred and forty-three profit-making facilities were investigated, and 258 investigations have now been completed.

The audit findings, including some supplied by the Department of Health's Bureau of Audits and Investigations, identified over $63 million in cost overstatements of proprietary homes (Hynes 1978c, p. 1). Since investigations of fifty-two facilities have yet to be completed, the final disallowances will probably be somewhat higher.

This figure was based on unaudited cost reports of more than $1.3 billion and resulted in the claim that "approximately five cents of every Medicaid nursing home dollar during this period subsidized fraud" (Hynes 1979, p. 7). This however, appears to be a somewhat inflated figure.

First, the OSP estimated that of the $63 million in overstated costs occurring during the period, $42.6 million represented Medicaid overpayments to proprietary facilities. Table 4.3 summarizes the nature of these overpayments.

Second, total state Medicaid expenditures to nursing homes and health-related facilities from 1971 to 1977 amounted to about $5.1 billion. The OSP investigation was restricted to 343 proprietary nursing homes and about $1.3 billion in unaudited cost reports.

Third, OSP claims for each disallowance would still have to withstand administrative and judicial appeals designed to protect the rights of the operator.

Audit disallowances were initially turned over to the Health Department for recoupment. The Health Department might or might not agree with the OSP's calculations. In a number of cases, these audits were returned to the OSP because of what was felt to be incomplete documentation. The operator was entitled to an administrative hearing. A new Division of Audit Appeals was set up to process such requests. After evidence was presented on both sides, the hearing officer would make a recommendation that might involve supporting the full amount, rejecting it, or compromising somewhere in between. The Commissioner of Health would then make a final determination, based on the recommendations of the hearing officer. If not satisfied, the operator could extend the appeal in the courts through an Article 78 procedure that is available to an individual who seeks redress from the administrative actions taken by a government agency.

No recoupment was attempted until after these proceedings were complete. If there was a relatively large sum involved, the operator had little to

Table 4.3

Cost Disallowances by Reimbursement
Category for Proprietary Nursing Homes
1969–75 Cost Reports.

Reimbursement Category	Disallowances (% of total)
Operating expense disallowances	43.59
Equity disallowances	33.55
Property disallowances	22.71
Patient days	.15
Total	100.00

Source: Hynes 1978c, p. 18.

lose by extending the appeals process. Once this process was complete, instructions concerning the adjusted rate for a particular facility for the years in question would be forwarded to the local social service commissioner. It was then the duty of the local commissioner to go to his files and determine how many Medicaid days of care had been reimbursed to that facility for that particular year. The local commissioner was then to calculate the actual amount owed to the state by the facility and work out arrangements with that facility for recouping the money. The money could be paid in a lump sum, installments, or adjustments in the current rate. If one of the first two methods was adopted, the local commissioner was responsible for appropriately allocating federal, state, and local shares.

This last stage proved to be a particularly weak link. Local social service departments varied greatly in their ability to cope with recoupments. In some cases, the records could not be found. In others, the local commissioner concluded that the amount of money to be recovered was not worth the money and staff time required to process the recoupment. Others faced more immediate pressures such as timely payment to providers and could not divert their energies to this area. One respondent reported a situation in which an operator, frustrated with the delay in receiving reimbursement from the Department of Social Services, placed a patient in a wheel chair in the parking lot of the nursing home and called the social service commissioner to pick him up (Respondent 46 1978). No matter how the money was recouped, there was no guarantee that it was not obtained at the expense of the patient rather than at that of the operator. Some of the apparent footdragging by local social service departments may have been for this reason. In 1979 the process was streamlined. The state Health Department recalculated certified rates of payment for the homes and forwarded these rates to the local social service commissioners. Since the actual dollar amount owed could be calculated from the adjusted cost reports, and the rate adjustments needed to recoup the amount owed could be calculated with a fairly high degree of accuracy, it is puzzling that this approach was not adopted initially. Respondents questioned about this were also puzzled. The problem appears to lie in the difficulties of coordinating two state agencies that have overlapping responsibilities. The Department of Social Services has, since the beginning of the Medicaid program, been designated as the single state agency responsible for it. However, the Health Department, at the time of the implementation of the Medicaid program, assumed responsibility for setting Medicaid reimbursement and enforcing standards. Recurring legislative and administrative attempts to consolidate the Medicaid program in one or the other of these agencies have not eased coordination problems between the two.

Strengthened by a court ruling (*Solnicik* v. *Whalen,* 1978 App Div), the Health Department began recoupment by adjusting rates before the appeal process was begun, while providing for the initiation of appeal hearings within thirty days of the rate adjustment. This served to speed recoupment and, probably, to both shorten the appeal process and give the Health Department more leverage in negotiating any compromise with the facility.

Before this resolution, the OSP had reached its own conclusions (Hynes 1978c, pp. 23–24):

> However, the administrative process was so vague and ill-defined that it turned out to be practically interminable. And, this was only the first hurdle to be overcome. Beyond the administrative process loomed the prospect of lengthy court challenges to the Department's administrative conclusions. Assuming the State could prevail there, local counties would still have to act, each on its own . . . All these delays cost a facility operator absolutely nothing. Any objection, no matter how frivolous to the State's findings could be argued on both the administrative and the court level.

In 1977 the OSP was authorized by the Attorney General to institute civil suits to recover Medicaid payments. A supplementary budget was obtained and in September 1977 a special Civil Recovery Unit went into operation. Of the $42.6 million of Medicaid overpayment as of 31 December 1979, $39.6 million in alleged overpayments was available for recovery, as indicated in Figure 4.5.

The recapture of the remaining $3 million was still pending completion of investigations. As indicated in Figure 4.5, relatively little has been recaptured. Civil cases involving $10.9 million have been forwarded to the Department of Health for recapture because, "where the value of the audit

Figure 4.5

Recoverable Medicaid Funds as of December 31, 1979:
by the Office of the Special Prosecutor, $28.7 Million;
by the New York State Department of Health, $10.9 Million

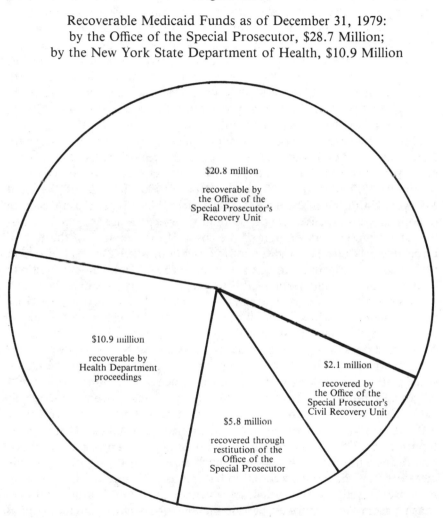

$20.8 million

recoverable by
the Office of the
Special Prosecutor's
Recovery Unit

$10.9 million

recoverable by
Health Department
proceedings

$2.1 million

recovered by
the Office of the
Special Prosecutor's
Civil Recovery Unit

$5.8 million

recovered through
restitution of the
Office of the
Special Prosecutor

Source: New York State Office of the Special Prosecutor 1980.

finding is under $25,000 ... the amount in question *would not justify the expense of a lawsuit.*" [Hynes 1978c, p. 25 (italics added)]. It is unclear, assuming that an operator chooses to contest, whether this would in fact be any less costly. As of December 1979, $5.8 million has been recaptured or pledged in criminal cases involving fraud. Two operators, Bernard Bergman and Eugene Hollander, accounted for $3.5 million of the $5.8 million. Some civil recoveries involve overpayments where fraud cannot be proven. As of December 1979, only $2.1 million had been pledged or collected. Almost all of these civil recoveries resulted from negotiated settlement. Because of delays created by attorneys representing facilities, only two court settlements, totaling $398,000, have been awarded (Respondent 76 1980). This leaves an additional $20.8 million theoretically available for recapture by the Civil Recovery Unit.

Thus, a four-year intensive investigation involving a combined Health Department and OSP audit force of over 300 professional auditors and a more than two-year intensive effort at civil recovery have succeeded in recouping $7.9 million as of 31 December 1979. The cost of the Civil Recovery Unit itself is about $300,000 per year, but it is perhaps inaccurate to compare this expense with the amount recovered, since the operation of this unit represents only a part of the costs. If the activities of the Health Department's Bureau of Audits and Investigation, which the OSP utilized in their own investigations, are added, total costs would be substantially higher. While it would be impossible to assign an actual cost upon which all parties would agree, no one is arguing that such audit and recovery activities pay for themselves. In spite of all the initial rhetoric concerning the rate of return for investment in additional audit and investigatory staff, recovery does not appear to be a money-making proposition. Nor is it fair to judge the performance of recovery activities on this basis. Except for the fabled speed traps in small rural towns, law enforcement and criminal prosecution have never been profit centers in state or municipal governments. Their value must be argued more in terms of their deterrent effect, an exceedingly difficult concept to measure. As mentioned in Chapter Three, costs reported in 1975, in the midst of the investigations, apparently dropped significantly in relation to reimbursement received in 1974. Other possible measures must be more anecdotal in nature, as evidenced by the following response, secretly tape-recorded, of a vendor salesman to a hospital purchasing agent's request for a 5 percent kickback: "I can't do it in the hospital industry anymore, the boss won't let me. I can do it in hotels and restaurants, but the Hynes Commission is all over the place" (Respondent 75 1980). In the experience of New York State, anyone who says that fraud and abuse units will directly pay for themselves in terms of the money they are able to recover is guilty of false advertising. Their value depends mainly on what they are able to deter. There was no consensus among respondents about the relative magnitude of those numbers.

What is particularly striking, as the dust begins to settle, is not how much proprietary operators were able to embezzle from the Medicaid program in this environment of relatively little audit or enforcement capability, but how little theft could actually be proved. Conviction for criminal fraud requires that proof of guilt be "beyond a reasonable doubt." In a civil recovery case only "clear and convincing evidence" is required. However, balancing out the difficulty in proving intent in fraud cases and the indeterminate status of a number of investigations, a 1 percent figure would seem a conservative estimate of the amount of the fraud. While some of the cases have yet to be completed, recoveries in others have involved civil cases. About 1 percent of the total amount reimbursed to proprietary facilities between 1971 and 1977 has been either pledged or recovered.* Even if one uses the OSP's estimate of 5 percent fraud, it does not appear to be disproportionate to disallowances found in other kinds of institutions and agencies from which HEW purchases services. An HEW audit of the New York State Department of Health itself for some $36 million in contracted services between 1971 and 1976 produced initially over $1 million in disallowances (2.7 percent). A substantial portion of this was related to disagreements concerning the cost-sharing of the Medicare and Medicaid survey activities for nursing homes. Harvard University's School of Public Health fared even worse in a recent audit. Out of $37 million in HEW grants and contracts awarded to the school between 1975 and 1978, $2.5 million (7.7 percent) were identified as being inappropriately charged (Brazda 1979, p. 3).

There is no evidence to suggest that overstatement of costs is any more of a problem with the proprietary nursing homes than with any other agency or institution from which the state or federal government purchases services. Ironically, the only real challenge to this conclusion comes from respondents representing proprietary nursing home interests, who, hostile to the stance taken by the OSP, have berated the competence of the OSP audit, investigative, and legal staff.

The relationship between the Health Department and the OSP appears to have been most strained over issues concerning audits and recoveries from homes. There were two groups performing similar functions and competing with each other for budgets. A certain degree of bureaucratic rivalry was inevitable. The *Third Annual Report* of the OSP announced, "to date, this

---

*Based on pledges or recoveries of $11 million as of January 1980 on review of $1.3 billion in unaudited cost reports from proprietary homes.

office has submitted 136 audits of proprietary nursing homes to the Health Department which represent the audits of 31% of the nursing home beds in the State. These reports identify overstated nursing home operating costs of $28,593,609" (Hynes 1978a, p. 21). This figure was used to support the earlier prediction of the OSP "that a Special Prosecutor audit of all 367 proprietary nursing homes in New York State for the period 1969–1973 could identify Medicaid overcharges approximating a minimum of $70 million" (Hynes 1976, p. 20).

From the perspective of some Health Department staff, the proprietary operators were not the only parties guilty of overstatement. An internal memorandum requested by the director of the Office of Health Systems Management expressed frustration concerning the OSP figures. They claimed "no one now in the OSP could provide definite details on how that particular number [$28,593,609] was generated" (New York State Department of Health, Office of Health Systems Management 1978, p. 1). It was also claimed that many of the totals were arrived at by Health Department audits. Their projected recoveries were far less optimistic. OSP audits for seventeen years, with potential recovery of $110,000, have been certified and approved, and OSP audits for eighteen years have been sent to the Bureau of Audits and Investigations for release to providers for possible revision on appeal of $106,000. A conservative value of $10,000 per year of audit can be based on these returns. The Health Department estimated that the actual value of the OSP audits would not be likely to exceed $4 million (New York State Department of Health, Office of Health Systems Managment 1978). That projection has proved to be incorrect, but so, apparently, have those of the OSP.

A memorandum of understanding worked out under the auspices of the Senate and the Assembly finance committees enabled the OSP to receive 120 additional auditing positions in the spring of 1976. The legislature had initially balked at budgeting these additional positions for the OSP in the midst of the state's fiscal crisis. Their resistance was characterized in the press as a reprisal for OSP investigations and indictments of legislators. Members of the finance committee, however, maintained that the decision to eliminate these positions had been made at the staff level. They restored the positions to the OSP budget with the requirement that an agreement be worked out between the OSP and the Health Department so that duplication of functions would be avoided. The new auditing staff would be shared between the Health Department and the OSP and would eventually revert to the Health Department.

This face-saving device has not been trouble-free. There was conflict over what was perceived as common turf. There were also problems because of the different function and emphasis of their audits. The Health Department's Bureau of Audits and Investigations was oriented toward recovery through rate recalculations. Such audit disallowances would have to be carefully specified and documented to withstand appeals by operators, which would further slow recovery. The orientation of the OSP audits was successful identification of fraud. Inevitably, buck-passing resulted. In some cases, the audits turned over to the Health Department by the OSP were returned because of lack of documentation and for recomputation of the rate. Given what the Health Department perceived to be inflated projections of recoveries, it was not eager to recalculate these rates and lay itself open to accusations of mismanagement by the OSP. Submission of other OSP audits to the Health Department was delayed, pending the outcome of criminal proceedings. There is a six-year statute of limitations on recoveries based on audit findings. The delays of criminal proceedings threatened recovery of some of the overpayments.

There are a number of loose ends concerning the management of audit and recoupment efforts that have yet to be sorted out. One major question has to do with the relative efficacy of the OSP's civil recovery route and the Health Department's procedures for recoupment. In 1979 the Health Department instituted a program of recovery by adjusting the rate of reimbursement. Such recovery, as long as it assures a timely hearing process for the facility, can be instituted immediately; it need not wait for the final resolution of appeals. Further, the state, in such an administrative hearing, presumably has a clear tactical advantage. The burden of proof rests with the operator. He must prove by submitting additional evidence, that the disallowances made by the Health Department auditors are incorrect. In a civil proceeding, the burden of proof rests on the state, which must provide evidence in court that an operator overstated his costs. Article 78 court appeals are supposedly limited to those claiming that due process was not afforded an operator in the Health Department administrative hearings. There are, however, a number of other avenues that could be pursued in obtaining such judicial review. Operators could prevent immediate recoupment by obtaining an injunction against the Health Department. Lawyers representing the industry prefer to defend their clients in a civil suit rather than to represent them in an administrative hearing, acknowledging the advantage that such a procedure gives the state (Respondent 34 1979). The inability of the Health Department to begin quickly has proved to be a problem, due to limited staffing.

In any event, the process of recovery has not been as simple as was suggested by those advocating additional auditors in the early 1970s or as was projected at first by the OSP. The cost of additional staff for field audits has not been the only cost. One must also act upon the audit findings, and that has proved to be a Pandora's box.

The apparent confusion between the roles of the OSP and the Health Department audit staffs appears to be creating other problems. While the Health Department audit staff expanded rapidly in 1975, prior to OSP's efforts to eliminate the backlog of proprietary audits, it is currently being reduced by attrition. The backlog of audits is growing again. As of November 1979, the backlog in the Bureau of Audits and Investigations has grown to over 2,000 audit years (Respondent 48 1979). The objective of auditing cost reports prior to reimbursement is becoming unrealistic. Given the experience to date, it would appear to be far more efficient to deter fraud and abuse before it takes place rather than try to recoup losses afterwards. That would ideally involve audits before reimbursement, as well as vigorous investigations and prosecution of fraud.

Patient Abuse

Patient abuse was a focus of OSP activities from its inception. A small unit was set up to handle such cases. The OSP's New York City patient abuse unit currently consists of three lawyers and six investigators. Two of these investigators are registered nurses and five have had experience as police officers. The unit also has access to additional investigative staff as the need arises. One attorney in each of the regional offices is responsible for patient abuse cases. During the first four years of operation, over 500 patient abuse cases were investigated.

The number of investigations undertaken has approximately doubled as a result of the implementation of the patient abuse reporting statute (Public Health Law 2803-D) in April 1978. This development will be discussed in detail in Chapter Five.

These investigations resulted in only five indictments for patient abuse and one indictment for unsafe and unclean conditions. Of these indictments, one conviction has been obtained, two cases have resulted in acquittal, two are still pending, and one has been dismissed and is currently on appeal (Respondent 11 1978). The one conviction involved a nurse who struck a patient in the face, causing a serious bruise. A case dismissed by a lower court involving an aide who had forced a patient to swallow his own feces was reversed by the Appellate Division. A trial resulted in a hung jury and the lower court then dismissed the case in the interests of justice.

In general, patient abuse is exceedingly difficult to prove. Families of a patient are rarely in a position to have first-hand information. Abuse usually involves patients who are the least mentally or physically capable of presenting evidence. Often the actions take place without witnesses. Most incidents involve aides and other untrained staff. The OSP has come to recognize the impossibility of approaching the patient abuse problem strictly from the point of view of prosecutions. Among its other recommendations, the OSP has pushed for greater training and licensure control over these employees.

The benefits of OSP activities in regard to patient abuse must rest in the deterent effect (Respondent 11 1979):

> People in the industry are very afraid of us. They are not afraid of the Health Department. When we go out and investigate possible incidents involving assaults on a patient, they know we are not out there to give them a deficiency. If there is an assault complaint, we are out there in a couple of hours with a camera ... If you know an aide has been involved in the abuse of a patient, but can't prove it, you can still read them the Miranda warning and question them. The chances are they will think twice before they will hit a patient again.

Certainly OSP activities have caused greater awareness of the problem. Record-keeping concerning incidents has no doubt improved even if much of this is of the defensive variety. There has also been a change of attitude concerning cooperation with the OSP. Backing from the OSP gives an operator leverage in dealing with unions that might object to his firing an abusive employee.

Perhaps more significantly, the OSP has been a new actor in the regulatory policy formulation process. It was directly involved in the task force that developed regulations concerning the 1977 patient abuse reporting statute. It has been involved in making recommendations to expand that legislation to cover hospitals and to tighten some of the loopholes. Sending initial drafts of the new nursing home code to the OSP stimulated forty pages of comments and, eventually, its full participation, along with some of the New York City consumer groups, in the process of developing the code. In a sense, the OSP has evolved into a lobby countervailing that of the industry associations. It has served to make the process of developing the code more open and public and has also shaped its character. The greater specificity, accountability, and precision of efforts to alter legislation and regulations is a response to the OSP's needs in terms of criminal prosecution, a concern that had not been so consciously addressed in the regulation development process before.

Public Misconduct

An assumption of improper political influence underlies most of the early reports in the press and statements by Stein, Cuomo, the Moreland Commission, and the OSP.

How else could substandard care be ignored for so long? How could some nursing home, real estate, and construction ventures produce so much conspicuous wealth so quickly? How could the use of Medicaid funds for personal luxury items by operators be ignored for so long? According to the Watergate ethos, there had to be a bagman with a payoff somewhere. Attention was focused by the Stein and Moreland investigators on a number of public officials.

Those who shared this dubious limelight included: T. Norman Hurd and Robert Douglass (top aides to former Governor Rockefeller), C. Daniel Chill (then counsel to the Assembly minority leader), John Marchi (New York State Senator), Louis J. Lefkowitz (Attorney General), and Stanley Lowell (former Deputy Mayor of New York City). Accusations reached all the way to the governor's office. Former Governor Rockefeller was accused by the Moreland Commission of permitting the existence of an atmosphere in which corruption was allowed to run rampant (Hess, 21 March 1975). Former Governor Wilson was called to testify before Stein's Temporary State Commission on Living Costs and the Economy regarding two meetings he had with Bernard Bergman (Hess, 27 March 1975).

The two prominent political figures subjected to the most intensive scrutiny were Albert Blumenthal, Democratic leader of the Assembly, and Stanley Steingut, speaker of the Assembly.

Blumenthal was indicted on perjury charges related to his testimony before the Stein and Moreland commissions. This testimony concerned a meeting in April 1971 at the Park Crescent Nursing Home. The home was a Bergman facility and was facing problems of licensure and certification. Other participants in that meeting disagreed with Blumenthal about the content of the meeting and Blumenthal's role in it. Blumenthal had earlier labeled the indictment "unfounded and outrageous ... so motivated by political sensationalism that it'll fall on its face" (Hess, 6 December 1975). In March 1976, in an attempt to plea bargain, Bergman pleaded guilty to the bribery of Blumenthal in a case involving manpower training subcontracts. As a result, Blumenthal was indicted for receiving unlawful fees and payments. He described Hynes as a "prosecutor gone mad, willing to bribe a confessed thief" (Hess, 12 March 1976).

Rumors were rife during March 1976 in political circles concerning the other politicians that Bergman might implicate. Stein, then campaigning for the Democratic senatorial nomination, said in a speech, "They'll have to hold the next session of the legislature in the Tombs" (*New York Times,* 13 March 1976).

All charges against Blumenthal were dismissed shortly afterwards. Justice Aloysius J. Melia was critical of the handling of the case by the special prosecutor. In dismissing the indictment, the acting Supreme Court justice "excoriated the special state prosecutor, in language seldom seen in judicial opinions, for violating several well-established legal rules designed to protect the rights of defendants"(Goldstein, 18 April 1976). The OSP failed to overturn the dismissal on appeal in December 1976. The Appellate Court, less critical of the OSP, reached the following conclusions (*People* v. *Blumenthal*):

1. An indictment charging defendant, a member of the Legislature, with a violation concerning unlawful fees and payments, receiving a reward for official misconduct in the second degree, receiving unlawful gratuities and nine counts of perjury was properly dismissed. While defendant assisted a named individual in convincing the New York State Department of Health to license said individual to operate a nursing home located in defendant's Assembly District, defendant did not receive or demand any unlawful emolument or promise of compensation.

2. Perjury counts alleging false statements before a legislative commission were properly dismissed since the District Attorney of New York County had not been superseded and it was not a matter for the Special State Prosecutor.

3. A perjury count in connection with statements concerning receiving a promise was properly dismissed inasmuch as no such violation was found.

4. A perjury count having to do with what defendant understood was properly dismissed since what defendant's understanding was is an operation of the mind.

5. A perjury count charging that defendant said that he did not "vouch" for a certain nursing home whereas he allegedly did "vouch" for that home was properly dismissed. Whether particular statements constitute "vouching" is a matter of interpretation of the statements and the word "vouch."

6. While two perjury counts come close to being statements of fact, it accomplishes little for justice to subject defendant to a trial on a negligible aspect of the charges without substantive counts and with the surrounding counts dismissed.

Blumenthal resigned from public life shortly afterwards, claiming vindication.

Heated disagreements took place between legislators and the OSP in 1976. Several Health Department and legislative staff members expressed high regard and affection for Blumenthal and bitterness concerning his treatment by the special prosecutor. During March of 1976, the request by Charles Hynes for additional auditors and staff, and funding of $2.3 million was deleted at the last minute by the legislature prior to submitting the request to the governor. Hynes' allegations that the decision was made in a meeting of the Democratic and Republican leadership was vehemently denied by the legislators, who insisted that it had been done at the staff level. Blumenthal indicated that Hynes had "slandered not only the entire leadership of the legislature, but me in particular" (Greenhouse, 18 March 1976, p. 45). Senate Majority Leader Warren Anderson expressed annoyance at "the pressure tactics employed by Mr. Hynes to embarrass the legislature into restoring the money" (*New York Times* 20 March 1976, p. 17). Anderson indicated that Hynes' decision to "go to the press" with his complaint about the deletion was an "indication of an attitude I abhor in any prosecutor" (*New York Times* 20 March 1976, p. 17). Hynes later retracted his earlier statement and described the incident as a "breakdown in communication." Anderson raised serious questions about the apparent duplication of functions in the Health Department and the OSP in terms of auditing, and questioned the advisability of placing auditing staff in an agency whose temporary nature would result in recruitment difficulties. With some concessions, the OSP-budgeted positions were reinstated in mid-April, at the same time Blumenthal's indictment was dismissed.

Although Steingut was not indicted by the OSP, his activities received extensive scrutiny by the press, the Moreland Commission, and the Temporary State Commission on Living Costs and the Economy. He initially was alleged to have told an assistant of Stein not to investigate homes owned by "my friend, Bernard Bergman." This was denied by Steingut. However, a state Health Department memo indicated that Steingut had interceded for Bergman. Stein alleged that Steingut had sought to block the investigation of homes belonging to Bergman. The Grand Brokerage, Inc., of which Steingut is co-owner, handled several insurance accounts for nursing home owners Bergman and Schwartzberg. Four thousand dollars was moved from Bergman interests into a Steingut-controlled campaign fund. One Bergman nursing home contributed $500 to a Steingut-controlled campaign fund and then applied for Medicaid reimbursement on the grounds that the money had been a legal fee. He was also said to have been involved in an attempt to reverse a Health Department decision not to grant Bergman a license to open the Danube Nursing Home. In retrospect, there does not appear to be any qualitative difference between Steingut's response to requests of a constituent and long-time political supporter and that of any other legislator. He had responded, however, to someone who was to become the focus of intense investigations. Steingut, who became speaker of the Assembly, lost a bitter Democratic primary election in 1978 for his seat from Brooklyn. The issue of the Bergman connection was again raised, and Andrew Stein, then borough president of Manhattan, actively campaigned against him. The unwritten but generally adhered-to code of state politicians prohibits such incursions onto one another's turf.

The activities of key Health Department staff also received intense scrutiny. As one Health Department official put it, "I came out smelling like a rose, but I didn't enjoy the process of getting there" (Respondent 45 1979). Some of these officials had not been insulated from attempts at influence by the operators. One official received a diamond necklace for his wife in the mail, a gift from an anonymous benefactor. In another instance, on Christmas morning in 1971, a man proceeded to unload three gift-wrapped boxes on the porch of another Health Department official. He waved and yelled, "Merry Christmas," and sped off in his car. The boxes were a case of 12-year-old scotch, a case of Canadian Club, and a case of French champagne. Often, influence attempts were more subtle and tailored to the special weakness of an official. For example, one operator just happened to drop by and just happened to have a pair of front-row seats to a sold-out championship basketball game that he wasn't going to be able to use; he wondered if the official, an avid fan, would mind taking them off his hands. In none of these cases did officials succumb to temptation. Offers involving women and sexual favors also took place, according to one respondent, but they were refused.

Attempted payoffs for the right decisions were usually only hinted at, as suggested by the following reported conversation (Respondent 45 1978):

> Lawyer representing a nursing home interest: Hey, you'd better be careful. Word is that there is $25,000 on the street for the right decision.
>
> Official: Wow. Thanks for warning me, I'll put a note in the record to protect myself.

Intensive investigations by the OSP could turn up no instances where decisions had been criminally influenced by such efforts or, indeed, any instances where officials had responded illegally to these approaches.

Prior actions by the Health Department, however, in the bright light of scrutiny by the OSP, could be made to look peculiar. A year-long investigation of a particularly controversial lease and sale to Broome County of the Willow Point Nursing Home and Health-Related Facility raised a variety of questions about the actions of public officials. Broome County had negotiated a lease with an option to buy that was highly profitable for a local group of investors before construction of the Willow Point Nursing Home. The lease agreement, signed in November 1967, resulted in the construction of a 162-bed skilled nursing facility which opened its doors in February 1969. The timing proved opportune, since the Health Department reimbursed the full cost of the $20,695-a-month lease. It was only in 1970 that captial reimbursement ceilings began to be imposed on new public facilities. The earlier trust in cost figures provided by public institutions, however, appeared to be misplaced in the case of Willow Point. The county nursing home administrator had entered into an agreement secretly with the investors before approaching the county. The final arrangement proved very beneficial for the partners. In addition to netting $15,000 a year, after the payment of the construction and equipment loans, they appeared to be guaranteed a minimum profit of over $100,000, as a result of the county's option to buy (Hynes 1978b, p. 7). Apparently encouraged by the financial success of the endeavor, the investors entered into an agreement with the county concerning the development of a 180-bed health-related facility as an adjunct to the newly leased and operating nursing home, with a $36,409 per month five-year lease and an option to buy at what turned out to be over $1 million more than the actual construction and equipment costs. The lease assured the investors of a profit of $53,000 per year, after paying off the building and equipment loans, with no additional investment of their own. The health-related facility was opened in November 1972. This time the county got burned. The Health Department's Division of Health Economics had developed ceilings for arms-length rental situations in order to protect the Medicaid program from paying for fat, sweetheart leases. The ceiling in this case was $287,000 annually as opposed to the $436,904 that had been agreed to by Broome County. In other words, the county would have to absorb the $149,905 difference.

The county appealed for a waiver from the ceiling and asked for the assistance of their state senator, Warren Anderson, in facilitating action on their appeal. In August 1973 the annual rate was revised to $324,000 retroactive to the date of opening, thereby reducing the county's annual loss to $112,905. Faced with these costs, as well as upcoming renewal of the lease for the nursing home that would involve an increase tied to the New York City Consumer Price Index, the county decided to exercise its purchase option. The price of the skilled nursing home and health-related facility combined was approximately $7.2 million. This was substantially more than the amount the Health Department's records showed as the total project cost (approximately $4.7 million) or the appraised value obtained by the Health Department ($5.3 million). The Health Department was thus faced with a second fait accompli with which they found it extremely difficult to live. While the actual reimbursement costs were less than those that had been approved for the lease arrangements, $239,233 per year as opposed to $537,346 for the leases on both facilities in 1973, there was no reason that this excessive purchase price should be honored in terms of Medicaid reimbursement. Broome County could have been left holding the bag in a situation they had created. The Health Department's notions of reasonableness, given an impossible situation in which they had been at least a passive participant, eventually resulted in an agreement for a thirty-year, rather than the standard forty-year, depreciation arrangement and acceptance of the $7.2 million purchase price as a basis for reimbursement. The relationship between the state Medicaid program and a county government is not comparable to that of the state and a private entity operating a nursing home because the county shares equal financial responsibility for the program with the state. If both the federal and state shares of the costs were denied, the financial viability of the third partner could not be a matter of complete indifference. These subtleties were ignored in the OSP cross-examination of the former director of the Division of Health Economics, as indicated by the following (Hynes 1978b, pp. 40–41):

Q. And my question to you is if on March 1st you accept a figure after an appraisal of $5.3 million when the sale is an accomplished fact — it is not a question [that their] purchasing is anywhere contingent on what you people are going to do?

A. I understand.

Q. I understand you gave [Broome County officials] no advance commitment?

A. Absolutely.

Q. Correct me if I am wrong, but $5.3 million for depreciation purposes as opposed to the rental arrangement is cheaper by $2 million than $7.2 million . . .?

A. Correct.

Q. So would you not agree that it is illogical, to say the least, to justify $7.2 million as opposed to $5.3 million on the theory that it is cheaper than the rental — the bottom line being that $5.3 million is cheaper than $7.2 million?

A. I agree one hundred percent.

Q. How did you go from $5.3 million to $7.2 million as far as what you recognize as the base for depreciation for this home — assuming that both are cheaper than the rental arrangement? That's the question.

A. I think I can only answer that one way, and that is when we determined that it would be cheaper than what we [were] paying, we accepted it.

A cross-examination of the assistant director brought this response (Hynes 1978b, p. 44):

Q. $5.3 million after a fait accompli; the sale is consummated, irrevocable on the part of Broome County, is cheaper than what you were reimbursing them under the lease arrangement?

A. Correct.

Q. My question: Do you recognize now, and did you recognize then, that $5.3 is at least $2 million cheaper than $7.2?

A. Of course, yes.

The special report by the OSP on Willow Point concludes, "to this day, [the officials'] actions remain a very expensive mystery for the taxpayers of New York State" (Hynes 1978b, p. 45).

If the actions of the Health Department officials were a mystery, the actions of the OSP with regard to this case, from the perspective of some Health Department and industry respondents, were equally mysterious. The OSP has brought a civil recovery suit against the now-retired official, the county officials, and the developers, for $1.3 million. It is peculiar, if not unique, to sue a private citizen for recovery of the cost pertaining to decisions he made as a public official and from which he received no financial benefit. From the OSP's perspective, it was necessary to name the former official in the suit in order to prevent the developers and local officials from claiming that what they had received had been fully consented to by the state. Some Health Department and industry respondents, however, questioned the attention devoted to the Willow Point case by the OSP. To them, the case appeared to have political overtones, as did the earlier investigations of legislators.

Actually, the political mudslinging had begun before the OSP was created, and it was one of the OSP's charges to investigate these allegations. The OSP did not initiate them.

In any event, after four years of investigation, the OSP concluded that the evidence for prosecution of public misconduct "was just not there" (Respondent 81 1978). Indeed, there is no mention of improper policial influence in the 1978 report of the OSP. The public legislative ethics bill, originally proposed by the Moreland Commission in 1975 to prevent legislators, Health Department employees, or firms with which they were associated from doing business with nursing home operators, was never passed. While no convictions directly related to nursing homes resulted from these investigations by the OSP, all respondents did indicate that the presence of the special prosecutor had produced a new climate of self-consciousness and caution among Health Department officials and legislators.

Conclusions

Respondents, depending on the interests they represented, disagreed on what conclusions could be drawn. While these investigations and prosecutions have been and will continue to be fraught with controversy, some underlying themes can be extracted.

The implementation of the OSP represented a bruising collision between professional subcultures that have been, with the exception of malpractice suits, quite insulated from each other. Health-related professionals have largely adopted the values of the medical profession, which emphasize autonomy, professional courtesy, trust, and accommodation. They found themselves subjected to a legal-investigative effort that not only shared none of these values, but also created an adversarial process that required formal, detailed documentation and an underlying distrust of the motives of anyone connected with nursing homes.

Some nursing home operators and other health-related professionals found the adjustment difficult. In the initial stages of the investigations, some investigators are reported to have questioned possible witnesses late at night with handguns visible in holsters, inquiring about the sex lives of suspects. There were protests by operators. Some likened the atmosphere of fear generated to that created by the Russian KGB or the Gestapo. Paranoia flourished among proprietary operators in 1975.

Sometimes the OSP staff ended up spooking not only those whom they questioned, but themselves as well. According to one account, OSP auditors in one home had borrowed a calculator from the administrator and had begun to pore over the records of the home in an available room in the nursing home. When the administrator attempted to contact them over the nursing home's intercom system in order to retrieve the calculator, the auditors were startled. An angry and what was seen as a threatening phone call ensued from the regional attorney accusing the home of "bugging" his auditors (Respondent 80 1976).

On the other hand, the lawyers and investigators in the newly created OSP, few of them with any prior health-related experience, were appalled by the seemingly informal expenditure of large sums of money and by the apparent lack of control over standards. This informality hindered their own efforts to investigate and prosecute, particularly in terms of reimbursement of capital costs and recovery of overpayments.

There is a greater degree of mutual adaptation between the OSP and others in 1980 than there was in 1975. Operators, for example, have learned to use the OSP for help in removing abusive employees. The organization and the leadership in the Health Department has shifted away from the traditional public health disciplines and toward legal and financial skills more compatible with the orientation of those in the OSP. The OSP has moderated its earlier investigative approach. Fear generated by OSP investigations has assumed more realistic dimensions.

This clash in subcultural values and orientations, of course, was not an insulated philosophical debate; it had real consequences in terms of political power, budgets, and positions in the state bureaucracy.

Caught in the backlash of Watergate, the regulation of nursing homes

was a political, not merely an administrative, issue. Careers of state politicians were both launched and prematurely ended by this issue. The state
Health Department lost its low-profile professional character, and the
future of its leadership was tied more closely to that of the governor.
Whether the OSP was able to maintain the independence and political
neutrality it asserted was essential to its mission or not, it was inevitable that
others would interpret its actions in political terms.

Perhaps even more intense was the rivalry for resources that erupted
within the state bureaucracy itself. The Health Department's Bureau of
Audits and Investigations, the Department of Social Services' Fraud and
Abuse Unit, the Welfare Inspector General, local and federal prosecutors,
and the OSP all competed for budgets, staff, and recognition. It is not surprising that each was critical of the activities of the others, that claims of
their own effectiveness tended to be exaggerated, and that cooperation and
communication among them was less than perfect.

Table 4.4 gives the chronology of investigations, scandals, and reform
efforts in New York nursing homes and their predecessors. A superficial
review might lead one to conclude that, since 1824, nothing has really
changed but the packaging. The same allegations of excessive costs, substandard conditions, fraud, and political impropriety continued to surface
at regular intervals. The cycle of concern and neglect follows a familiar
pattern (Slater 1970, p. 15):

> Our ideas about institutionalizing the aged, psychotic, retarded, and infirm
> are based on a pattern of thought that we might call the "Toilet Assumption"
> — the notion that unwanted matter, unwanted difficulties, unwanted complex-
> ities and obstacles will disappear if they are removed from our immediate field
> of vision. We throw the aged and psychotic into institutional holes where they
> cannot be seen. Our approach to social problems is to decrease their visibility:
> out of sight, out of mind ... When these discarded problems rise to the
> surface again — a riot, a protest, an exposé in the mass media — we react as if a
> sewer had backed up. We are shocked, disgusted, and angered, and immedi-
> ately call for the emergency plumber (the special commission, the crash
> program) to ensure that the program is once again removed from con-
> sciousness.

Yet, just as the political cycles of increases in Medicaid expenditures for
nursing homes have been dampened as result of increasing cost controls,
similar shifts have taken place in overall controls, lowering the public
threshold at which a new cycle of investigations and reform efforts would
be triggered. As suggested in Figure 4.6, the emphasis on controls in terms
of all programs for the indigent shifted first from essentially undifferentiated local political control to more specialized institutions with profes-

Table 4.4

Chronology of Investigations and Reform Efforts
Related to the New York Nursing Home Industry.

Year	Action
1824	State investigations into poor laws and their administration reported excessive costs, inadequate administration, and insufficient care.
1838	A state Assembly investigation found no separation of inmates with regard to age, sex, sickness, or sanity. All were housed in the same overcrowded rooms.
1840	Local justices of the peace in charge of outdoor relief for the indigent were accused of being too lenient in the granting of assistance to their own communities, while causing the county to absorb the costs.
1845	General turmoil over policies related to outdoor relief led to the replacement of the Commissioner of Almshouses.
1856	Survey by the state Senate found deplorable conditions in local almshouses. The Senate recommended that separate homes be created for children and the insane, that persons impoverished through no fault of their own not be confined to almshouses, and that a state agency to supervise almshouses and other institutions be established.
1860	State almshouses were organized into a Department of Public Charities and Corrections, with four commissioners.
1867	The Board of State Commissioners of Public Charities was created.
1873–1878	Almshouses in New York were involved in the Boss Tweed political scandals concerning the distribution of aid. All relief was halted in 1874–75 as a result of scandals.
1875	Children were finally excluded from almshouses.
1890	The mentally ill were finally excluded from almshouses.
1894	The first licensure legislation was enacted by means of an amendment to the New York State constitution which required private facilities caring for children to be certified by the state Board of Charities in order to be eligible for payments from local governments.
1926–1927	National exposés were published, discrediting almshouses.
1947	A woman on relief was discovered to own a fur coat, thus causing the "fur coat scandal," which eventually led to the dismissal of the Commissioner of Welfare. A city Department of Welfare was organized.
1958–1962	Investigations exposed misconduct in proprietary homes in New York City, leading to allegations of fraud and substandard conditions, follow-up investigations, and reform efforts.
1974–1980	Nursing home exposés were published. Reform efforts were begun.

Sources: Thomas 1969, Somers 1969.

Figure 4.6

Qualitative Shifts in Patterns of Control of Health Care
Providers

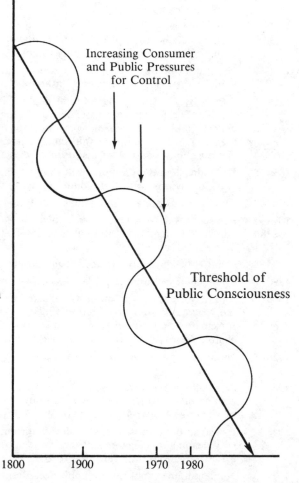

Undifferentiated:
Local political
control of all
institutions for
the indigent

*Professional-
normative;*
Creation of
specialized health
care institutions;
delegation of control
to professional
licensure and
accreditation bodies

*Bureaucratic-
utilitarian:*
Delegation of
professional standards
enforcement to public
agencies; increased
public role in
financing, thereby
producing more
restrictive interpretation
of standards
and more precise
cost-related payment

*Adversarial-
coercive:*
Clear conflicts
between public
agencies and
professional groups
emerge; pressure for
consumer rights,
punitive sanctions,
and cost competition

Pattern of Control

Increasing Consumer
and Public Pressures
for Control

Threshold of
Public Consciousness

1800   1900   1970 1980

sional controls in the form of licenses and accreditations. A second shift resulted from more centralized forms of reimbursement. Increasingly more bureaucratic controls were imposed over standards and reimbursement. Finally, concern over the increasing costs of those services and over the rights of the actual consumers of those services appears to have produced a third shift, one toward more punitive sanctions and a more adversarial relationship between the regulated and the regulator. It is this new environment that nursing homes and other health care providers must begin to adapt to in the 1980s. Chapter Five will review the impact of emerging consumer pressures on that adaptation.

Chapter Five

Enhancing Consumer Controls

"What about the patient?"

That refrain echoed throughout the efforts to tighten professional standards, sharpen reimbursement controls, and assure more aggressive prosecution. These efforts, as indicated in the three previous chapters, were often blunted, at times hollow, and sometimes self-serving. The need for these efforts at all, however, underscores the insulation of nursing homes from consumer pressure. Nursing homes are more insulated than other providers of health care services and are far removed from the comforting calculus of self-interest that, at least in economic theory, assures the responsiveness of providers through the interplay of market forces. Patients can exercise some degree of choice in selecting a physician. Elderly patients, however, often have little choice of a nursing home. Nursing home beds, as a result of certificate-of-need controls, are in relatively short supply. Consequently, patients and their families, particularly Medicaid patients, often have little choice but to take the first available bed. Although hospitals are also subject to certificate-of-need constraints, these constraints have been relatively less effective. The "surplus" of acute care beds often creates direct, aggressive competition between hospitals for patients or, more often, for physicians to fill beds in particular services. Nursing homes do compete for a small segment of the market, the private pay patients. Since charges paid by such patients are often substantially higher than the cost-based reimbursement for Medicare and Medicaid patients, private pay patients are more desirable. In some cases, private patients in nursing homes actually subsidize the care of Medicaid patients in much the same way private patients have historically subsidized medical care for the poor (Posner 1971, p. 29; Grimaldi 1980). Private pay patients, however, account for less than 15 percent of all New York nursing home revenues. Many proprietary and public facilities serve Medicaid patients exclusively. In addition, hospitals are predominantly voluntary community institutions, which, at least in theory, are more responsive to consumer interests. In contrast, 54 percent of nursing home beds in New York State are owned by private business. Thus, nursing homes are not only less influenced by competitive market forces than hospitals, but are also, because of their ownership, less responsive to consumer-public interests.

Added to this insulation, of course, is the nature of nursing home patients themselves. They are often seriously ill and hardly in a position to act as advocates for themselves. Nationally, 58.3 percent are described as suffering from senility, and another 18.6 percent suffer from mental illness; 88 percent do not have spouses upon whom they can depend to assist in assuring that their needs are met (U.S., Department of Health, Education, and Welfare 1977, pp. 5–6). Many, particularly Medicaid patients, do not have other relatives who can effectively look after their interests. Even if the relatives are actively involved, they are handicapped by lack of information about alternatives to nursing homes; they may not even know that there are alternatives. Unlike the consumer who returns the rancid milk to the grocery store, the nursing home patient is a captive of the institution. Fear of reprisals for complaints about staff or conditions is often well-founded. Nursing home patients are also the least likely to recover to the point where they can escape from such dependency. Nursing homes are usually the patient's last home. The bulk of discharges are either because of death or transfer to a hospital where death may follow shortly afterwards.*

Recognition of the need for other methods of patient protection, methods that involve broader consumer, constituency, or advocacy groups, predated the creation of the modern nursing home. In 1872 the New York State Charities Aid Association organized visiting committees made up of philanthropic private citizens who were to call upon every charitable institution in the state (Thomas 1969, p. 26). Shortly thereafter, the association was given the legal right to inspect any almshouse in the state. This group was successful in bringing about many changes. Its efforts were instrumental in outlawing the placement of children in almshouses and contributed to the development of specialized state facilities for the care of the mentally ill. The work of the association set the stage for the New York Public Welfare Law of 1929, which mandated relief to the poor in their own communities and served as the prototype for current public assistance programs. Ironically, the success of the association contributed to the dwindling of its influence and that of other social welfare advocacy groups. Its efforts resulted in the development of specialized institutions and contributed to the emergence of professional controls, which eventually insulated these facilities

---

*A crude survey of discharges from New York City homes revealed that only 6 percent of proprietary and 2.5 percent of voluntary nursing home patients actually succeeded in "escaping"—that is, in being discharged on their own recognizance (Respondent 4 1980).

from such voluntary advocate groups. The passage of the Public Welfare Law in 1929 resulted in drastic curtailment of the role of public and voluntary charitable institutions in the care of the indigent through its restriction of payment of funds to the indigent in institutional settings. Private boarding homes, which were outside the purview of advocate organizations and restrictions, assumed an increasing role in the care of the indigent elderly. These facilities eventually evolved into the proprietary nursing home sector. Local commissioners of public welfare negotiated contracts with such private institutions for the care of their elderly indigent charges. The commissioners also assumed responsibility for the licensure and standards of these facilities.

The state Health Department, recognizing the magnitude of the task it assumed in 1966 when it gained responsibility for nursing home licensure and surveillance, attempted to rekindle constituent or voluntary advocate group efforts in this area. The New York State Retired Teachers Association, which boasted of its ability to execute a visitation program for their members in every county in the state, was approached by the state Health department. Efforts to involve this group in a nursing home visitation program, however, never materialized. The association viewed retirement income and housing as far more salient issues for their members. It was also, no doubt, difficult to mount much enthusiasm from their members for a volunteer visitation program. Whereas it was thought that an elderly group could most closely identify with nursing home patients, the visits proved to be particularly stressful to many members. The last thing most of the retired teachers wanted to do was visit nursing homes. It takes particular strength of character to volunteer to work with seriously ill individuals, especially for those who may be filling their beds shortly. Efforts to involve the New York State Association of Retired Persons were unsuccessful for similar reasons, as were efforts to involve directors of senior citizen clubs in an advocacy role. The Health Department did, as a part of these early initiatives, recruit retired persons to survey a sample of twenty nursing homes. Deliberately unguided, the potential consumers were asked to describe their impressions of each home. Their methods of assessment differed significantly, as might be expected, from that of Health Department inspectors, federal standards, or the state nursing home code. They tended to be far more critical, and they focused on the quality of life for patients in the homes rather than on medical aspects. Crises involving conflicts between the state, the federal government, and operators over the enforcement of the Life Safety Code began in 1972 and ultimately absorbed all of the energy of Health Department staff in this area; it precipitated the abandonment of efforts to involve consumer constituent groups (Respondent 9 1978).

In 1974 the increased press coverage and investigatory attention focused on the nursing home industry in New York State highlighted a number of perhaps predictable problems associated with the protection of the rights of patients. They included misuse of patient funds, physical abuse of patients, and the continued operation of substandard facilities that have been described in previous chapters. This chapter will focus on various strategies that were adopted to end the almost complete insulation of the industry from the involvement and influence of consumers and advocate groups.

The problem of assuring an effective role for consumers and advocate groups may be more pronounced in the nursing home sector, but it is no different from that of involving consumers and advocate groups in the health sector as a whole.

An often overlooked article of faith in a democratic society is that the process by which decisions are arrived at is more important than the decisions themselves. If one shares, or at least partially shares, this belief, then perhaps the most emotion-laden, intractable, and perplexing problem facing the health sector is how to assure an adequate consumer voice in decision-making. No matter where critics of the health sector fall along the political spectrum, the lack of such a voice has generally been identified as a cause of the ills they describe as afflicting the system. These ills include uncontrolled, escalating costs, gross distortions in the overly specialized array of services, fragmentation, geographic maldistribution, gross discrepancies in the quality of care provided, and consumer alienation, as evidenced by the rising number of malpractice suits. This perception has been shared, at least vaguely, by Congress, which has imposed requirements for consumer representation on federally funded neighborhood health centers, mental health centers, health systems agencies, and some hospital rate review and rate-setting commissions. These efforts to assure greater consumer involvement have not been embraced with great enthusiasm by the health sector and have sometimes generated a good deal of controversy. Generally, these initiatives have not lived up to the expectations that served as their rationale.

A multifaceted effort to assure more effective consumer involvement began with the New York State nursing home reform efforts in 1975. The results of these efforts have provided some lessons for involving consumers more effectively in health care regulation and policy in the future.

Changes

There were at least four strategies that could have been adopted to assure greater nursing home responsiveness to consumers. All four were attempted, beginning in 1975.

Disseminating Information to Consumers and Their Families

The cheapest strategy in terms of public expenditures was simply to provide more and better information to the general public concerning conditions in nursing homes. This would, in theory, force nursing homes to be more responsive. Consumers would become more knowledgeable about their options, and this would create more competition among homes. Such greater visibility would also, it was thought, force regulatory agencies to be more responsive to consumers. Critics felt that what they viewed as the conspiracy of silence between regulators and the industry needed to be broken. As a result, the following steps were taken in 1975.

1. More aggressive use of the news media—The traditional low-profile role of the Health Department ended in 1975. The department began releasing to the press monthly reports of facilities with significant operating deficiencies.

2. Posting inspection reports—The nursing home reform package that became law in August 1975 required the conspicuous posting in each facility of a summary of the deficiencies identified in the most recent survey.

3. Grading facilities—The nursing home reform package also required that the Health Department develop procedures for weighting the importance of its various standards. It further required the development of not less than five categories for rating homes in terms of the quality of care provided. Those ratings would also be conspicuously posted within the facility. It was the intention of the legislature that this rating system would serve as a guide for consumers on nursing home services in much the same manner as, for example, the American Automobile Association's evaluation of restaurants (one to five stars) aids travelers.

Making Standards More Responsive to Consumers

Until 1975, the state code for nursing homes had largely served as a vehicle for upgrading the status of nursing homes and those professionals who worked within them. Emphasis was shifted in 1975 to focus on the responsiveness of the institutions to their patients. This was an attempt to deflect the barrage of criticism aimed at the Health Department and the industry by Stein's group, the Moreland Commission, and the press.

1. Patient's bill of rights—A patient's bill of rights was included in the 1975 legislation. This, in itself, simply provided state codification of federal Medicare regulations. The facility was required to inform the patients of these rights by conspicuously posting the policies and procedures related to

the bill of rights and to develop in-service training for staff to promote compliance with the requirements of the law. Section 414.14 of the New York State Code, Title X, outlines a number of specific patient rights including: the right to information about services and charges, to adequate and appropriate medical care, to transfer or be discharged, to voice grievances, to manage one's own financial affairs, to freedom from mental and physical abuse and from chemical and physical restraints, to security of one's personal possessions and confidential treatment of personal and medical records, to freedom of association, and, if married, to assurances of privacy during visits and permission to share a room if both are in-patients. Any violation of such rights that was reported to the Department of Health would be investigated. Homes were required to provide copies of this bill of rights to patients and their families.

2. Efforts to develop a more responsive code—In the fall of 1976, spurred by criticism on all sides, the Health Department organized a task force to start developing a new code. The initial objective was to simplify the code, but pressure from the newly emerging nursing home advocacy groups and the OSP changed the objective to that of making the code more responsive to consumers.

Improving Consumer Access to the Redress of Grievances

Simply improving the rules governing nursing home operations would have little impact if no effective means of redress existed. No inspection program could monitor the care a patient received on a day-to-day basis. Consumers, their families, and their advocates had to be assured of a rapid response to complaints. A variety of tactics was developed to assure this responsiveness.

1. Investigation of complaints by the Health Department—Procedures were initiated to investigate complaints and to assure that patient rights were protected. A hotline was established for complaints, and its telephone number was posted in facilities. A patient advocate was designated in each of the regional Health Department offices. All complaints required field investigation.

2. Volunteer ombudsman program—In 1977, with assistance from a grant from HEW's Administration on Aging, the state Office on Aging began to set up a volunteer ombudsman program. In cooperation with local community agencies, volunteers were trained to serve as advocates for nursing home patients and to make regular visits to the homes.

3. Patient abuse reporting law—Neither relatives nor volunteer advo-

cates were in the best position to observe the day-to-day treatment of patients. Only those working in a facility could be expected to be familiar with their daily treatment. The patient abuse reporting law (Chapter 900 2903-d) tried to tap this resource. Licensed professionals, under possible penalty of loss of license, were required to report any potential incidents of patient abuse to the regional office of the Health Department. An on-site investigation of each report by regional office staff was required within forty-eight hours.

4. Class action suits — If administrative remedies were unsuccessful or too cumbersome, a class action suit could be initiated. According to the 1975 legislation, a facility that deprived patients of rights or benefits provided for by state law or pursuant to contract was liable for injuries suffered by the patient as a result of that deprivation. A minimum for compensatory damages was set at one-quarter of the daily Medicaid rate per patient for each day that the patient's injury existed. Punitive damages could also be assessed against the facility if it was found to have been in willful or reckless disregard of the lawful rights of patients. These payments would be exempted from consideration for Medicaid eligibility and need not be applied toward payment of medical services. The court could also award attorney's fees. Controlling persons within the institution were made personally liable in order that, if the facility were bankrupted by such a suit, the court might extract payment from their personal assets. Insurance for such a liability was not a reimbursable expense.

Enhancing the Psychological and Legal Senses of Ownership

Critical to establishing a sense of consumer control, if not the reality of this control, is the perception of ownership. Ownership in this context refers to the broader psychological perception that the facility or services belong to the consumer, that they are his or her nursing home, hospital, and so on. This overlaps the more narrow legal definition of ownership, but it is distinct. For example, some labor unions have established Health Maintenance Organizations, but the rank and file members do not perceive them as their own. On the other hand, some small voluntary and even proprietary hospitals in rural communities are clearly perceived as belonging to that community, even though the board and governance of the facilities may not formally reflect this perception.

There has been an erosion in both the legal and psychological senses of ownership by consumers and their constituent groups in health care during this century. By far the greatest erosion took place in the emerging nursing home sector after 1929, when restrictions on assistance to public and voluntary institutions spurred the development of the private nursing home sector. This initial step was compounded by the creation of a standards-generating process that came with Medicare and Medicaid. It forced the closing of the "Ma and Pa" operations and created the chain operations. This disengagement from a consumer ownership made the proprietary nursing home sector a particularly easy political target. Some of the initial proposals of 1974 suggested the elimination of the proprietary sector altogether.

The scandals of 1974 and 1975 facilitated the creation of a number of nursing home advocate groups, primarily in New York City. A variety of groups, including Friends and Relatives of the Institutionalized Aged, Community Action Resources for the Elderly, Legal Services for the Elderly Poor, and Coalition of the Institutionalized Aged, sprang up to act as watchdogs of the channels established for the protection of patients. Pressures on operators of substandard facilities led to the appointment of receivers and the eventual closing or sale to new owners. In a number of cases, community groups were organized to take over the facilities.

Results of Disseminating Information

One of the Health Department's efforts to disseminate information to consumers and their families was to issue press releases identifying facilities with significant operating deficiencies. These press releases became more infrequent after the first six months in 1975 and were discontinued by the end of 1976. They were reportedly a source of friction between operators and the Health Department. One operator reportedly called up, incensed that his facility had been lumped with what he regarded as really lousy places. The Health Department itself was far from consistent in its definition and reporting of facilities with significant operating deficiencies. These inconsistencies and the apparent lack of confidence in the results, as well as pressure from the homes, led to a discontinuation of the press releases.

The summarized inspection reports continued to be posted, as required by the 1975 law, along with the plan of correction. Most informants agreed that, except in extreme cases, they were of relatively little value to a prospective consumer or his family. The summaries focused on code deficiencies, many of which were not directly related to patient care or easily interpreted by a consumer.

The rating system, described in earlier chapters, went through a number of modifications. No one expressed much confidence in the ratings as a tool for consumers. There were too many inconsistencies across regions. Eighty-eight percent of the nursing homes in 1978 were clustered in the "good—state" category; the ratings failed to discriminate effectively between facilities. There was not much enthusiasm for the rating approach within the Health Department. No effort was made to develop a consumer handbook listing the ratings; consequently, they were unavailable to an individual shopping for a home for an elderly relative.

It appears that the rating system, as a consumer tool, never received a fair test. The procedure developed was methodologically flawed and overly subjective. In several ways it went against the grain of those responsible for its implementation. First, if the rating system was really meaningful and did discriminate between facilities, certificate-of-need restrictions would result in the relegation of a certain proportion of patients to facilities with inferior ratings. These would most likely be Medicaid patients. Acknowledgement of such a two-class system of care might have unpredictable and probably unpleasant political consequences. Second, if the Health Department did accurately rate a certain set of homes as inferior, part of its mission was to make sure that high standards of care were assured. Why wasn't it doing its job? Clearly, there was a conflict of interest.

Results of More Responsive Standards

The patient's bill of rights in the 1975 legislation helped underscore the dissonnance between the existing standards and the assurance of the basic rights and dignity of patients. Existing standards patently failed to address these issues. They focused on structural considerations, building standards, sanitation, staffing, documentation, and so on, not on the patient and the effect these issues might have on him as a human being. The professional model of regulation took the protection of those rights largely for granted, a matter of professional trust. That trust had been severely shaken in the nursing home sector.

In the fall of 1976, a task force was organized by the Commissioner of Health to develop a new code that would focus on performance and outcomes in terms of patient care and that would eliminate some of the burdensome paperwork. Drafts of these documents met red flags raised by emerging consumer advocate groups in New York City. The new code was interpreted as a watered-down version of the old one and a sellout to the nursing home industry. New York City groups, Friends and Relatives of the Institutionalized Aged, Legal Services for the Elderly Poor, and Community Action Resources for the Elderly, as well as staff in the patient abuse section of the OSP first demanded to participate in the development of the new code and then essentially took over the rewriting and revision process. Representatives of the industry remained relatively inactive in the process, which involved intensive work by these consumer groups during the summer of 1977. Up until this point, the development of standards and regulations in the health sector, often including the actual writing of them, had been heavily influenced, if not controlled, by provider associations. Now, perhaps for the first time, a coalition of consumer advocate groups controlled the development of the document that was to set the basic standards for nursing homes. Initially, there was a sense of exhilaration among the groups, for, as one put it, "he who controls the document, controls the outcome" (Respondent 10 1978).

The new code tightened the language and controls. Particular attention was given to the conditions under which physical and chemical restraints could be used, to the protection of the personal funds of patients, and to the transfer of patients. The resulting document probably increased, rather than decreased, the burden of paperwork on the operator, but it did succeed in more effectively protecting patient rights. The code was approved by the Hospital Review and Planning Council in the fall of 1977. It was never implemented, however. It became clear that, in order to be effective, the mini-maxi standards had to be repealed. The implementation of the new code without repeal of the mini-maxi provisions by the legislature would have been a hollow victory. No facility would need to comply with these standards. Predominantly Medicaid facilities would be least likely to comply. That repeal was not forthcoming. The nursing home associations lobbied effectively against it. They raised the issue of the cost of the new regulations. A figure of $50 million a year in additional Medicaid costs as a result of implementing the new standards was presented by the Health Facilities Association. The legislature and Division of the Budget were responsive to those concerns. A public interest auditing group assisted the New York advocate groups in contesting this figure, but no one could argue that it would not cost at least some additional money. The mini-maxi requirements remained in place, and the new code remained in limbo.

Much of the steam was lost by the consumer groups. Most of the original group of active individuals have left the movement, and some of the groups have become dormant. The effort invested in the code revision "undermined our resources for no return. It destroyed us" (Respondent 4 1980). The ad hoc coalition for a single, standard nursing home code, formed in 1977 and encompassing some thirty-five groups (including local consumer groups, the Gray Panthers, 1199, the OSP, the Office of the Aging, Friends and Relatives of the Institutionalized Aged, Legal Services for the Elderly Poor), however, continue to lobby for the passage of such legislation. Some interest in sponsoring such a bill in the 1980 session surfaced.

Results of Improving Access to Redress

In 1975 a statewide hotline was established for complaints, and individuals in the regional offices were assigned duties as patient advocates to investigate such complaints. Chapter 900 of the Laws of 1977 added section

2803-d to the Public Health Law, requiring the reporting of suspected abuses of patients by residential health care facility professional and non-professional personnel.This legislation provided an important impetus for investigating such complaints. The law required that licensed professionals report by telephone and, subsequently, by written report all incidents in which they have reasonable cause to believe that abuse, mistreatment, or neglect of a patient took place. Licensed professionals failing to make such reports would be guilty of unprofessional conduct and would be referred to the appropriate licensing board. The New York City consumer advocate groups and the OSP played a significant role in the development of the legislation. A task force set up to implement the legislation by developing the appropriate regulations did not neglect to include representatives from the New York City patient advocate groups, the state Office for the Aging, and the OSP, as well as nursing home providers.

Health Department patient advocates were required to investigate within forty-eight hours any complaint alleging abuse. Upper-grade regional Health Department personnel were placed on call for weekends and vacations. Reports of abuse were referred to the regional OSP offices. In cases where criminality might be involved, the OSP conducted the investigations, sometimes jointly with the Health Department.

Implementation of the new patient abuse requirements in May 1978 resulted initially in an almost tenfold increase in reports. The results of those investigations as of 1 January 1980 are summarized in Tables 5.1 to

Table 5.1

Status of Patient Abuse Reports Made to
the Office of Health Systems Management

	1978	1979
Number of abuse reports	529	1295
Completed investigations in abuse report year	397 (75.0%)	*
Completed investigations in subsequent year	132 (25.0%)	
Decision rendered in report year	237 (44.8%)	530 (40.9%)
Decision rendered in subsequent year	239 (45.2%)	
Sustained in report year	90 (17.0%)	240 (18.5%)
Sustained in subsequent year	117 (22.1%)	
Unsustained in report year	147 (27.8%)	290 (22.4%)
Unsustained in subsequent year	122 (23.1%)	
No decision rendered	53 (10.0%)	765 (59.1%)

* Category not included in 1979 reports.

Source: New York State Department of Health, Office of Health Systems Management 1978, 1979.

Table 5.2

Action Taken on Completed Investigations of Patient Abuse Reports

Nature of Report	1978 Investigations Completed in 1978					1978 and 1979 Investigations Completed in 1979				
	On-site visit and referral to OSP*	Accused and facility notified of findings	Follow-up visit and/or recommendation to facility	Referral to licensing board	Other (commissioner's order)	On-site visit and referral to OSP*	Accused and facility notified of findings	Follow-up visit and/or recommendation to facility	Referral to licensing board	Other (commissioner's order)
Inappropriate physical contact	134	136	11	6	1	486	515	206	15	0
Mistreatment	12	12	4	3	0	35	42	14	13	0
Neglect	81	84	11	7	0	217	233	90	33	0
Combination of above	10	10	0	0	0	31	41	14	15	0
Total	237	242	26	16	1	769	831	324	76	0

Source: New York State Department of Health, Office of Health Systems Management 1978, 1979.
* Office of Special Prosecutor

5.3. The average number of reported cases statewide per month climbed from about 75 in 1978 to about 100 in 1979. Of the 529 cases reported statewide in 1978, 207 had been sustained with 53 still under investigation as of 1 January 1980. Thus, in about 40 percent of the cases reviewed by the Health Department's central office, there appeared to be sufficient evidence to suggest that physical abuse, mistreatment, or neglect had occurred. The most frequent source of reports was registered nurses, followed by administrators. Physicians were the least likely of the licensed employees to report. Aides were most likely to be the focus of investigations, other patients the next most likely.

"Inappropriate physical contact" was the most common incident given in reports. The bulk of reports resulted in referrals to the OSP. Most involved notifying the accused and the facility of the findings, while a relatively small number involved referrals to professional licensing boards for possible disciplinary action. The patient abuse law limits reporting requirements to patients in residential health care facilities (skilled nursing facilities and health-related facilities). Efforts to extend the provisions of the patient abuse reporting law to hospital staff have so far failed.

The program faces a variety of administrative problems. As a result of the implementation of the law, the amount of time committed to patient advocacy has increased by 50 to 100 percent in the regional offices (Rensselaer Polytechnic Institute 1979, p. 105). Reporting itself has been subject to some abuses. In some area offices, staff complained that a disproportionate share of patient abuse complaints arrived from facilities late Friday afternoons, requiring weekend duty to meet the requirement of initiating an investigation within forty-eight hours. Some facilities that may have felt harassed by the inspectors apparently used the opportunity to return some of the harassment. Use of the hotline and allegations of patient abuse also rose during labor negotiations and strikes, sometimes in an effort to embarrass the institution. There is a recognition of the need for training Health Department staff in investigatory techniques and for developing a better understanding of the nature of the criminal justice system. Seminars were conducted at the state police academy in Albany for 270 persons on the Office of Health Systems Management staff during the summer of 1979 (New York State Department of Health, Office of Health Systems Management 1979, p. 1). An earlier report on the Health Department's patient advocate program operations was highly critical (American Jewish Congress and Community Action Resources for the Elderly, 1977). There were substantial delays in investigating serious criminal and possibly life-threatening allegations. There was also lack of follow-up on complaints. Sometimes a protective attitude toward the homes caused investigators to judge the complainant rather than the merits of the complaints. How independent

Table 5.3

Completed Investigations of Patient Abuse Reports

Person Involved		Licensed employee										Nonlicensed employee										Anonymous		Total
		Administrator		Registered Nurse		Licensed Practical Nurse		Physician		Other[1]		Aide		Orderly		Patient		Family		Other				
		Total	Sustained	Total	Sustained	Total	Sustained	Total	Sustained	Total	Sustained	Total	Sustained	Total	Sustained	Total	Sustained	Total	Sustained	Total	Sustained	Total	Sustained	
Submitter of Abuse Report	[N]	74	31	57	32	2	2	2	2	21	9	4	1	●	0	3	0	27	4	19	5	29	5	238
(1978 Cases[2])	[%]	31.1		24.0		.8		.8		8.8		1.7				1.3		11.3		8.0		12.2		100
Report	[N]	146	75	252	142	7	4	9	5	51	30	19	7	1	0	21	5	106	23	87	44	70	22	769
(1978–79 Cases[3])	[%]	19.0		32.8		.9		1.2		6.6		2.5		.		2.7		13.8		11.3		9.1		100
Object of Investigation	[N]	1	1	14	2	25	13	1	0	4	0	77	36	25	15	1	0	1	0	11	6	89	23	249
(1978 Cases[2])	[%]	.4		5.6		10.0		.4		1.6		30.9		10.0		.4		.4		4.4		35.7		100
(1978–79 Cases[3])	[N]	4	2	48	34	48	32	15	8	0	0	262	98	54	28	118	108	5	2	14	9	263	72	831
	[%]	.5		5.8		5.8		1.8		0		31.5		6.5		14.2		.6		1.7		31.6		100

[1] Includes balance of professionals mandated to report by Public Health Law 2803-d.
[2] 1978 cases reported and investigation completed in 1979.
[3] 1978 cases reported in 1978 but investigation completed in 1979, and 1979 cases with investigations completed in 1979.
Source: New York State Department of Health, Office of Health Systems Management 1978, 1979, 1980.

can a patient advocate be if his findings reflect not only on the facility, but the reimbursement mechanism, standards, licensure, and utilization review procedures? Pressures to further integrate the complaint investigation functions in the New York City regional office with the activities of the regular survey teams, which so far have been restricted, seem to beg this question again.

Beginning in 1975, New York received federal grants under Title III of the Older Americans Act for development of a volunteer ombudsman program. The intent was to use the state Office of the Aging to facilitate the development of local volunteer programs. The Moreland Act Commission at the same time recommended the establishment through legislation of a mandatory program for homes. This and the so-called legislative ethics bill were the two pieces of reform legislation that failed to pass. The ombudsman bill, although passed by the legislature, was vetoed by the governor, who felt it to be a duplication of other programs established to monitor nursing homes that year.

The lack of such legislation, however, has placed the volunteer advocate program at a disadvantage. The groups needed the cooperation of the institutions themselves in order to gain access to the patients' environment. In selling the programs locally to the nursing homes, the ombudsman programs have attempted to soft-pedal the surveillance function and emphasize the service that the program provides to the homes (that is, a friendly visitor to patients, a means of identifying problems before they become serious, assistance in the implementation of the patient's bill of rights, assistance in preparing clients for discharge, and so on) (Glanzman 1978).

The proprietary nursing homes were initially more willing to cooperate with the program than the voluntary and public institutions. The latter institutions had escaped with little damage from the exposés, while the image of the for-profit institutions had been tarnished. The proprietaries had little to lose through such exposure, and many welcomed it. Pressure for access could be increased by contacting citizen leaders and local politicians, as well as legislation if voluntary cooperation were not forthcoming. A model plan for the state-initiated local programs was developed in 1977 by the Community Council of Greater New York. The October 1978 amendments to the Older American Act provide that 1 percent of federal Title III(B) social services funds allocated to the state Office of the Aging be used for nursing home ombudsman efforts. This amounts to about $204,000 in the case of New York for 1980. As of January 1980, there were 12 local programs in operation and about 100 volunteers participating in long-term care facilities caring for 10,000 residents. Volunteers undergo a thirty-six-hour training program and then agree to volunteer four to six hours a week to visit patients in nursing homes and adult care homes. The program covered about 7 percent of the nursing homes in the state. The ombudsman has dealt with issues such as assuring physician visits, entitlement to benefits, and transfer. In one case, ombudsman-initiated efforts succeeded in obtaining a court order restraining the local department of social services from transferring a patient.

Experience to date has suggested that "the more professional the background of the volunteers, the less effective they may be as advocates." Those with professional backgrounds may have difficulty divorcing themselves from their former roles and tend to generate friction among the facility's professional staff (Respondent 16 1980). Rapid changes are expected in the program as it attempts to expand to cover all nursing homes and adult care facilities in the state and bring the program into compliance with the regulations governing the 1978 amendments to the Older American Act. In order to establish procedures to assure access to the ombudsman, as required by the law, the state Office of the Aging is working with the state Department of Health and the state Department of Social Services to change regulations concerning the patient's bill of rights. The state Office of the Aging is also working with the legislature to pass a bill that would assure access (Respondent 16 1980).

Opinions differ about the overall effectiveness of the volunteer ombudsman programs. The problems most frequently identified by the ombudsmen concern nursing care. These have included lack of attention to the personal hygiene of patients, delays in answering call bells, and the attitudes of nursing staff towards their charges. The next most frequently identified problems are food and nutrition—that is, the quality of the food, the lack of availability of snacks, and so forth. The state Office of the Aging reports that about 60 percent of these complaints are resolved within the facility to the satisfaction of the patients (Respondent 16 1980). Others identified with some of the advocate groups are dubious about the overall effectiveness of such a volunteer program. They point to the relatively high turnover of volunteers and question the ability of the program to deal with the tougher issues. In general, the nursing home operators have been supportive.

The 1975 legislation also encouraged class action suits on behalf of patients who were denied rights or benefits created for their welfare by law or by reimbursement contracts with facilities. Compensatory damages were to be set at one-quarter of the facility's daily Medicaid rate per patient for each day that the condition persisted. Punitive damages could be awarded where the facility's actions were found to have been willful or in reckless disregard of the rights of the patients. These damages were exempt from determination of Medicaid eligibility. There are also provisions for the payment of legal fees.

Despite this seemingly attractive invitation to litigation, no class action suits have been brought against nursing homes. Although at least one law-suit has invoked this section, there have been no reported decisions (Respondent 10 1980). Nationally there has been almost no activity in this area (Sullivan 1980). One major deterrent appears to be fear of retaliation. As long as the patient remains within the institution, overt and covert retaliation may occur. Since length of stay is prolonged, recovery is unlikely, and transfer to other facilities is restricted, the nursing home patient is, in effect, the hostage of the institution. Patients and their families may be fearful and reluctant to undertake such transfers, preferring known discomforts to the unknown. Also, nursing home patients, unlike other consumer groups, are unlikely to reap the rewards of investing the effort in and taking the risks of such action. The life expectancy of such legal actions would probably be substantially longer than that of many of the appellants. The New York experience is similar to the national experience. There have been fewer than half-a-dozen suits nationally (Respondent 10 1980).

The image of a group of Medicaid nursing home patients sipping piña coladas in deck chairs on a Caribbean cruise ship, enjoying the fruits of their class action suit at the expense of an indifferent or avaricious nursing home operator, remains fantasy.

Results of Enhancing the Sense of Ownership

There have been shifts in the sense of community-consumer ownership. This is reflected in the involvement, for the first time, of consumer advocate groups in the development of legislation and regulation concerning nursing homes. The new code, although stalemated, involved substantial input by the New York advocate groups, particularly in the areas of use of chemical and physical restraints, management of the personal funds of patients, and the transfer of patients.

Advocate groups played a particularly important role in issues related to the transfer of patients. If the patients or their families are to develop any sense of psychological ownership, they must be able to have a say in where they live and when they move. Injunctions have prevented patients from moving without adequate preparation in Rochester and in New York. The New York case is perhaps particularly significant since it appears to have triggered similar cases across the country. The Village Nursing Home in Greenwich Village had been operating under a waiver from the state in terms of square foot requirements per patient. According to this standard, the facility was overcrowded by about 100 patients. The state Health Department, in the aftermath of the nursing home investigations, refused to give any additional waivers or to adjust the home's per diem rate upward to reflect the increased fixed costs per patient until the facility's census was down to the acceptable level. Thus, it was in the owner's financial interest to move these excess patients as quickly as possible. The facility apparently attempted to transfer their patients in large batches. Ambulances, according to one respondent, began to queue up outside before some of the patients who were to be moved or their families had been notified (Respondent 10 1980). The Gray Panthers and Legal Services for the Elderly Poor received a temporary restraining order until acceptable procedures could be developed for the preparation of such a transfer (*Fields* v. *Berger,* 1975). A subsequent case (*Feld* v. *Berger,* 1976) reinforced the right of patients to notification and to access to utilization review records. The *Yaretsky* v. *Blum* (1979) consent judgment questioned the entire utilization review process and will have profound effects on utilization review and transfer procedures in nursing homes. Protection, including requirements for a fair hearing, should be provided to a patient who does not wish to transfer from a facility. The ruling will make it difficult to transfer any patient from a facility against his will.

Advocate groups were also active in the development of patient abuse reporting legislation. The legislation was developed and its regulations largely written by a coalition of individuals in the New York City advocate groups. They have served as a countervailing influence on the regulatory process. There are, of course, serious limitations to their effectiveness. They operate on a shoestring. At their peak, four of the more active groups, (Friends and Relatives of the Institutionalized Aged, Community Action Resources for the Elderly, Legal Services for the Elderly Poor, and Coalition of the Institutionalized Aged) had probably fewer than five or six persons participating full time. The advocate groups rely on uncertain or nonexistent budgets and volunteers. Without their alliance with the OSP on issues of common concern, their efforts would probably be less effective. Although some success has been achieved, the groups still, by and large, lack close ties with the constituency they claim to represent. These groups have not reached the point where they are perceived by most nursing home patients or their relatives as the protectors of patient interests. They may be able to gain leverage through the press, but not through collective action by their purported constituency. Finally, the technical nature of many issues, the lack of access to information, the bewildering complexity of the regulatory process itself, and the need for constant pressure to get information mitigated against their effectiveness. What they have been able to achieve is impressive, given the array of financial, legal, and information sources with which they often find themselves in conflict. That effectiveness is as much a reflection of the lack of sense of ownership of nursing homes by the general public as it is of the organizing abilities of the advocate groups.

The state Health Department's preference for voluntary group ownership of nursing homes was given added impetus after 1975. As indicated in Figure 5.1, the proportion of new proprietary beds to voluntary and public beds in the state system began to shift after 1966. In 1966 over 80 percent of the new homes opened were proprietary, while in 1977 the number of new proprietary homes opened had dropped to zero. During this period, the bulk of nursing homes closed, 70 percent, were proprietary.

The 1975 legislation provided for two forms of receivership that may have assisted in facilitating this shift. Voluntary receiverships (New York

Figure 5.1

Increase in Number of Nursing Home Beds
in New York State, 1966–78

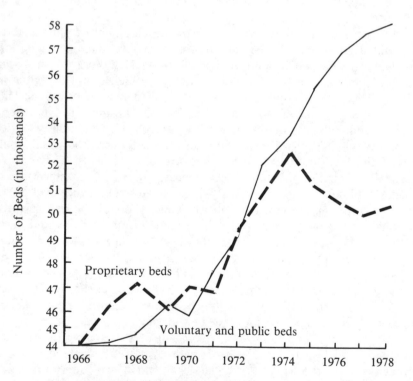

Sources: Dunlop 1979; Hynes 1976, 1977, 1978a, 1979; New York State Department of Health 1980.

[Public Health] Law. Article 28. Sec. 281.1) may be initiated at any time at the owner's request and may be created by the Health Department under conditions that are acceptable to both parties. Involuntary receiverships (New York [Public Health] Law. Article 28. Sec. 2810.2) may be issued upon the determination that operational deficiencies in the facility demonstrate substantial violation of federal and state law or regulations, other conditions dangerous to life, health, or safety, or a pattern of habitual violation of standards. The bulk of the receiverships, as indicated in Chapter Two, resulted from bankruptcy.

Starting in 1975, the Health Department compiled a "hit list" of homes that were either in serious financial difficulty or that provided poor care. The Department attempted to elicit interest in these facilities by voluntary organizations or community groups. Most of their efforts have proved unsuccessful.

The Village Nursing Home has become the major, if not the only, success story, although not as a result of Health Department efforts. The operator, faced with serious deficiencies, expressed a desire to get out of the business. The consensus of Health Department authorities was that the facility should probably be closed. The news sparked protest by one volunteer advocate, and the community organized efforts to prevent the closing. Many of the residents had strong ties to the Village, and opposition to their transfer was strong. Residents included Marian Tanner, Village philanthropist and prototype for Auntie Mame, and photographer Harry Fields. Legal Services for the Elderly Poor obtained a restraining order to prevent the transfer of patients. The Caring Community, a coalition of local religious and social groups, began a campaign to raise funds to buy the facility and "save our own people." Political leaders flocked to the cause. Congresswoman Bella Abzug and Congressman Edward Koch supported these activities. Former Attorney General Ramsey Clark headed a fund-raising drive that produced $200,000. The home was later visited by Rosalynn Carter, who expressed her support of the activities of the group. Mitchell Waife, director of Jewish Home and Hospital, served as receiver, and several of his staff assumed responsibilities at the Village Nursing Home. The home was eventually transferred to the community group. It obtained some waivers from the federal government of violations in the Life Safety Code and has proceeded with some fairly costly, but necessary, renovations.

Other efforts have not been as successful. A community group was formed to take over the Park Crescent Home, a bankrupt Bergman facility, but it has been hampered by an inability to raise funds, a lack of expertise, and a lack of the kind of cooperative relationship with the facility's court-appointed receiver that existed in the Village Nursing Home situation. Kings Harbor continues to be run by the Health Department while negotiations continue for the facility's takeover by a voluntary hospital. Another facility that was taken over by a community group from a convicted operator is in a questionable position, since the former operator still owns the facility and some of his relatives continue to work in it.

One major problem in terms of transfers has been money. The capital cost reimbursement that the Health Department allows may be substantially lower than that which the former operator or receiver is willing to accept. Prior debts of operators (mortgage payments to banks and debts to suppliers resulting from the bleeding of the facility), also become issues. Some facilities, such as the Village Nursing Home, required substantial renovation if they were to remain open. Community groups usually do not have access to the needed financial resources, and voluntary institutions, faced with their own financial problems related to their own reimbursement levels, are cautious.

Another major problem is the lack of expertise among community groups. The legal, regulatory, administrative, and financial issues concerning such a transfer can be exceedingly complex. The necessary skills and experience are rarely present in local groups. Several possible methods of alleviating the problem have been considered. The statewide Community Aid Association developed a proposal for creating a technical assistance unit for such efforts. The creation of a quasi-public corporation by the Health Department that would provide teams to assume receiverships and then assist in the transfer of the facility to a community group has also been considered.

The money problems are more difficult to resolve.

Conclusions

The reform efforts were successful in producing some additional consumer control. Consumer advocate groups were effective in influencing some legislative and regulatory changes. Such participation by consumer groups did not exist before 1975. The year 1975 was perhaps a watershed in New York in terms of serious attention to patients' rights. The old almshouse assumptions and stigma that had been carried over into the Medicaid program were pushed into the background. New avenues for redress of grievances were opened up to consumers.

Two general problems, however, continued to hinder the effectiveness of consumer reform efforts. First, there were conflicts in the objectives sought by many of the groups. One objective was to enhance consumer control by improving their information, giving providers a clear financial incentive to be responsive to consumer preferences, and making the Health Department more accountable to consumers and the public. The underlying ideology was that of a free, competitive market in which consumers would dictate which operators survived. Nursing home care should be subjected to the same market forces as other economic goods and services. This ideology guided efforts to create for consumer use a rating system of institutions and to link that rating system to reimbursement. The other objective here was to increase public-community control and ownership of the system. The underlying idea was that such services, since they were publicly financed, should be publicly owned, or at least publicly controlled. This guided the creation of certificate-of-need requirements and the Health Department's efforts to find voluntary groups to purchase or serve as receivers for proprietary facilities. The uneasy coexistence of both ideologies in terms of long-term care in New York restricted the ability to assure either greater consumer control or greater public ownership.

Second, efforts to assure responsiveness to consumer grievances were similarly caught on the horns of a dilemma. If they were incorporated into the Health Department's responsibilities for regulating the industry, a certain amount of defensiveness was inevitable. Poor performance reflected on the Department's own effectiveness as well as on operators'. On the other hand, it was difficult for outside groups, such as the state Office of the Aging's volunteer ombudsmen, to act because they tended to lack the information, resources, and leverage needed to be optimally effective against operators.

These and other, more general problems will be discussed further in Chapter Six.

Chapter Six

Summary and Conclusions

The dust has begun to settle and it is time to sort out what has happened. This final chapter will summarize the changes that have taken place between 1975 and 1980 and suggest some questions these experiences raise for the health sector as a whole.

It is easy to get lost in the morass of details described in the previous chapters concerning each approach used to control nursing homes in New York State. These details mask the underlying similarities in the problems associated with the regulation of any part of the health sector. Nursing homes have evolved from the same undifferentiated public and voluntary charitable institutions from which the modern hospital has emerged. They have followed the same regulatory pattern as hospitals. That pattern of control reflects the shifts similar to those in the regulation of individual health professionals. Control has shifted from the local community to voluntary professional associations and then increasingly to bureaucratic agencies. The strains created by those shifts are creating an increasingly coercive, adversarial regulatory environment.

The New York experience with the regulation of nursing homes represents what sociologists refer to as an "ideal type," an extreme case, that throws into stark relief some of the contradictions inherent in the more subtle shifts that have taken place in the regulation of the health sector as a whole. It represents the extreme in terms of the magnitude, dominance, and rapid increase of public financing.

The next section will summarize the results of the changes that took place in the regulation of nursing homes in New York between 1975 and 1980. The section that follows will address the more general questions such a case study raises for the health sector as a whole. The final section will depart from the essentially descriptive purpose of this study and make recommendations.

Results

It might be easy to survey some of the wreckage of the past five years of activity in New York and glibly conclude that nothing happened. Indeed, each of the previous chapters detailed reforms and initiatives that met stiff resistance, frustration, compromise, and, in some cases, abandonment. Some of those abandoned initiatives deserved their place in the dustbin. Others did not. The first few years may have been too filled with inflated rhetoric and too many unrealistic promises, which later produced disillusionment. It is a mistake, however, to focus on what did not happen. While they were not all entirely to the liking of either reformers or industry advocates, many changes did take place, as outlined below.

Professional Standards and Surveillance

The standards and surveillance process moved away from the JCAH professional model to a more bureaucratic one. Efforts to develop a more outcome-oriented code were undertaken, and efforts to rationalize the surveillance process through a more phased, selective scrutiny that would emphasize outcomes were begun. The standard-setting and surveillance process became more tightly linked to reimbursement through such processes as management assessment. Surveyors began to assume two new roles, that of an industrial engineer concerned with efficiency and that of a legal investigator concerned with enforcement. Some nursing home administrators lost their licenses, and a few facilities were turned over to receivers as a result of substandard care. The dramatic growth in number of licensed nursing home beds ended in 1975, and the number of beds remained relatively constant during the next five years.

Reimbursement

Cost increases in Medicaid reimbursement were dampened for nursing homes. Total Medicaid expenditures for nursing home care were lower in 1976 and 1977 than they were in 1975. A large field auditing staff and legal staff were added to the Health Department to deal with the resulting administrative appeals and litigation. There was more homogeneity imposed on reimbursement of proprietary and voluntary facilities. Restrictions in capital cost reimbursement eliminated any remaining incentives for real estate speculation in nursing homes.

Criminal Enforcement

Criminal prosecution became a credible threat. An independent well-financed unit was established. While fraud was far less pervasive than the initial reform rhetoric suggested, fines and jail sentences were imposed. A new form of control, fear of criminal prosecution, became institutionalized in the health sector.

Consumer Control

Legislation and administrative mechanisms were adopted to protect the rights of patients. New advocate groups emerged and became actively involved in the development of legislation and regulations for nursing homes for the first time since the establishment of the Medicaid program. These attempts to enhance consumer control, however, had relatively little impact compared to the other changes that took place.

Remaining Questions

In spite of the accomplishments, one is left with a sense of discomfort. The changes are still too incomplete. It is unclear where we are and where we should be going. There are too many unanswered questions.

Perhaps the basic lesson of the New York nursing home experience is that solutions create problems. The initial efforts in the New York Medicaid program to assure access to nursing home care produced problems in the enforcement of standards and financial abuse. Efforts to control quality through stricter enforcement of standards produced cost problems. Efforts to control cost increases by returning to a more restrictive, more nearly charge-related form of reimbursement appear to again be raising concerns about lowering quality. Efforts to enhance market controls through rating systems and the linkage of ratings to reimbursement raised problems in terms of equity. On the other hand, insulation of health providers from market controls encourages inefficiency and unresponsiveness to consumers. There appear to be no real solutions, only fluctuating tensions between conflicting goals, interests, and values.

Recognizing this, one is faced with recurring dilemmas in design, management, and politics of regulation.

There appear to be at least three dilemmas in terms of the design of a regulatory system for health care providers.

1. To what extent should regulatory functions be centralized or decentralized? What role should the local community, the state government, and

the federal government play? The more centralized, rigid, unresponsive, and ritualized the regulatory process becomes, the less influence consumers have in the process. On the other hand, at what point in terms of local control does the lack of uniformity make external control meaningless?

2. To what extent should regulatory functions dealing with access, cost, and quality be integrated with each other, and to what extent should they function independently? Integration assures fewer overt public conflicts, but how important or healthy is that?

3. How much permeability is appropriate? How responsive should the regulators be to the regulated? On the one hand, a deaf ear will guarantee ineffectiveness, but, on the other hand, at what point does it become unclear who is controlling whom, and is that important?

Once the design questions are answered, there are at least three recurring problems in the day-to-day management of such activities.

1. To what extent does one encourage the development of a professional model or a more bureaucratic approach? A more professional model requires more individual judgment and probably can produce more flexibility in responding to individual situations, but to what extent does this subvert control by making enforcement in an adversary situation more difficult? The more bureaucratic the regulatory process becomes, the more it increases the following problems.

2. How does one keep the process from becoming more ritualistic? A certain amount of decay is inevitable. What can be done in terms of the reward structure and job design to prevent this?

3. How does one keep the regulatory process from becoming a training center for the industry it regulates? Is it important to avoid this? There is very rapid turnover particularly in the financial area. Positions outside are more lucrative. A similar phenomenon has been noted in the Internal Revenue Service. The resulting rapid turnovers often mean that those on the "outside" often know more about the system than those on the "inside."

The regulation of health care, however, is not just a detached exercise in efficient organizational design and management. It involves a political struggle for control. In this particular case study, who won and who lost?

Such questions have been the focus of concern in much of the literature on regulation. Different models make different assumptions about who the winners and losers will be (Noll 1975). The traditional public interest model of regulation assumes that the consumers are the winners and that an omniscient and disinterested bureaucracy serves their needs. At the other extreme, the capture model of regulation assumes that the regulated industry is the victor, that regulation is the creature of the industry, designed to create a legally enforceable cartel. A less simplistic, political-economic model of regulation appears, however, to more accurately characterize the events in this particular case. According to such a model, while regulators attempt to play the role of honest broker between consumer and provider interests their choices become distorted by limited information, limited resources, and political pressure. While providers have sharply focused interests concerning specific regulations, consumers' and the general public's interests are far broader, more diffuse and, therefore, are harder to identify in specific instances (McClure 1980). Hence, legislators and the regulators will inevitably respond to these unequal pressures. In general, regulators tend to be dependent on the industry for information, lack the resources for a sustained battle with the industry and have difficulty absorbing the political costs of decisions that have adverse impacts such as the bankruptcy of inefficient providers.

In spite of all these handicaps, the state regulators in New York were able to win some additional control. The nursing home exposés and the fiscal crisis of the state did succeed, at least initially, in focusing more general public attention on the nursing home industry. The state regulators gained greater control over expenditures. They succeeded in demonstrating the ability to cap gross expenditures, curb the growth of nursing homes, and to better assure the appropriate use of their funds.

The nursing home industry, in the longer run, however, also won. The investigations purged the industry of many embarrassments, while at the same time imposing limits on the arbitrary actions of regulators through reimbursement, standards and criminal enforcement. If the industry could complain about being handcuffed by overregulation, they could also take some satisfaction in imposing the same fate on the regulators. The nursing home associations were strengthened by additional staff and by the appearance of a more united front.

Consumers of nursing home services and their families, however, lost. This is not to say that the general public did not benefit from the greater control of expenditures nor that consumers did not benefit from the elimination of some of the more clearly substandard facilities or the control of some abuses. However, consumers had less control than they had in 1975. They faced a more complex state bureaucracy and a far more organized industry composed of larger, more sophisticated institutions. Both the bureaucracy and the industry shared an increasing preoccupation with their own financial viability. The strategy generally adopted of constraining costs through restriction of access to care, largely through certificate-of-need, works to the advantage of both the operators and the regulators but not, of course, to the advantage of the consumer (Feder and Scanlon 1980). It has increasingly fallen by default on the courts to protect the rights of the powerless consumer of nursing home services against such economic concern as evidenced by such cases involving patient transfers as *Field* v. *Berger* and *Yaretsky* v. *Blum.*

Prescriptions

The real problem posed by the New York nursing home experience, then, is not how public agencies can impose standards and cost controls on providers or how providers can survive the imposition of these controls. The real problem is, as a result of these struggles, how consumers can assure the responsiveness of these providers and public agencies and prevent further erosion of their own control. Consumer responsiveness and control cannot, it seems, be assured simply by adding more watchdogs and devoting more energy to better organizing consumer groups. If greater consumer control is a desired objective, basic structural shifts would seem to be required. Adherence to the four structural principles outlined below would seem to be useful in helping to restore some semblance of consumer control.

1. *Decentralization.* Decisions concerning the financing, licensure, standards, and planning of health services should be made at the lowest feasible level. Such decentralization helps reduce the power of professional and provider associations while making the public interest in particular issues less diffuse. It helps focus accountability rather than having it diffused through many layers of local, state, and federal bureaucracy. It has the potential of providing greater consumer input into the services provided, and greater responsiveness to individual situations. Standards, for example, take on an aura of unreality when filtered through many layers, each layer adding its own rigidity. The problems of one institution in Massachusetts illustrate the point (Bicknell 1977).

> State code at the time of construction of the new wing for an institution for the handicapped required that night lights be constructed in each room two feet below the ceiling. During construction the code was changed to require night lights two feet above the floor. The facility was told to correct what was now a code violation, a process that would be costly. All of the patients in this wing, however, were blind.

2. *Miniaturization.* Services should be provided in the smallest units feasible. Large institutions create centers of power that are more likely to be controlled by professional and institutional interests and are more likely to be insulated from consumer influence. In terms of hard nosed efficiency criteria, the rapid growth in the size of health facilities in the United States should probably be reversed.

Assessment of economies of scale in nursing homes and hospitals have produced ambiguous results (Ruchlin and Levey 1972, Feldstein 1979, pp. 177–86). This is true mainly because institutions of different sizes generally do not provide the same mix of services. The most efficient size is dependent on the standards imposed and the characteristics of the services required. The more elaborate the standards and services required and, indeed, the more complex the regulatory apparatus, the larger an operation one will need to be efficient. What, in fact, do we, as potential customers of these services, want?

> A group of nursing home operators at a conference were asked to describe their own facilities. Some described brand new facilities with elaborate recreational and physical therapy programs and over 300 beds. One facility was a thirty-bed operation run by a religious order. The home had a small garden, some chickens and a stream for fishing. The Sisters spoke with great affection and interest about each of their residents. At the end of the session the participants were asked to vote for the homes in which they would prefer to be a patient. The thirty-bed home of the Sisters was the unanimous choice. (Respondent 80 1976)

One might be willing to pay less attention to such preferences if there were more persuasive evidence of the efficacy of larger, more elaborate institutions in the care of patients. Indeed, some of the evidence suggests the reverse. There is extensive literature documenting the adverse effects of institutionalization and ways to counteract those effects (Ainsworth 1977, pp. 18–24). The majority of therapies and programs for the elderly residents of nursing homes, however, seem geared more toward adapting them to the institutions rather than toward other goals (Respondent 4 1980):

> A Health Department staff person, involved in a review of nursing homes, anguished over where to send her mother, who had fallen and broken her hip. Her mental condition had deteriorated in the hospital. There was minimal physical recovery and evidence of advanced senility. No one had much hope for her recovery. The daughter consulted with others familiar with nursing home care in the New York City area. Given the prognosis, they chose a forty-bed, nondescript proprietary facility near where the daughter lived, rather than one of the more high-powered voluntary facilities in the city.
>
> Six weeks later, the mother was walking and going out on luncheon dates with one of the male residents. Her mental facilities were restored and she appeared far happier than she had been for many years. The daughter's only concern was her mother's pending marriage. (Respondent 4 1980)

In the last analysis, the optimal size for a nursing home may well be one double bed.

3. *Desegregation.* Consumers should be provided health services in the

least restrictive, least segregated environment that is feasible. Separate facilities for the retarded, for the mentally ill, and for the aged chronically ill inhibit the development of a sense of social solidarity. Reducing the segregation between acute, chronic, and the "TAPS" (temporarily ablebodied persons) will prevent the fragmentation of consumer interests. It works against the creation of institutions where people who represent unwanted problems can be sent to be forgotten. It would seem reasonable to utilize some of the excess capacity in acute hospitals for long term care as others have suggested. (Vladeck 1980). Expanded home care programs fit into this objective and appear feasible for some nursing home patients (Demkowich 1979). A nursing home without walls program was created through legislation in New York in 1977, allowing Medicaid patients to stay in their own homes while receiving services. Nine pilot programs in various counties are in operation and are currently being evaluated by the federal government. There is reason for caution. Simply changing the packaging and the labels does not eliminate the segregation any more than the prohibition of payments for indoor relief in the 1934 Social Security legislation eliminated institutions for the elderly poor. Nor does simply moving psychiatric and nursing home patients into substandard boarding homes move one closer to achieving real integration.

4. *Reappropriation.* Services should be owned, to the largest extent feasible, by those who will be utilizing them. This provides the greatest potential for consumer and community control. In the beginning of this century, public and voluntary community group ownership was the almost exclusive pattern of ownership. It is a supreme irony that increases in public financing have served to erode public and voluntary ownership. The erosion of public and voluntary ownership needs to be turned back. That does not mean that one has to forego the alleged advantages of the proprietary sector. Competitively bid management contracts to proprietary firms could be utilized where efficiencies could be obtained while still assuring ultimate community control as has been advocated by some (Shulman and Galanter 1976).

The argument for each of these structural changes, in order to be convincing, would have to be developed at far greater length than is possible here. It is an argument not so much for any specific pattern of financing or design of services but for a change in the underlying assumptions. We have tended to confuse the enhancement of the power of professionals and managers with the solution of social problems. *The burden of proof should lie with any proposed arrangement for the delivery of health services that require centralization, larger units, patient segregation, or more attenuated community ownership.*

Perhaps we have reached a new watershed. The gradual shift from local community to professional, to state and federal control of health care has been a costly one. It has created a structure that may collapse of its own weight long before the immense gap between what exists and what is obtainable in health and health care for us is closed. In the process of solving problems we have created others. Perhaps, in that process we have lost sight of where we want to go.

References

Acton, J. P., and Newhouse, J. 1972. *Compulsory Health Planning Laws and National Health Insurance.* Santa Monica, Calif.:Rand Corp.

Ainsworth, T. H., Jr. 1977. *Quality assurance in long term care.* Germantown, Md.: Aspen Systems Corp.

Allison, G. 1971. *Essence of decision: explaining the Cuban missiles crisis.* Boston: Little, Brown.

American College of Surgeons. 1920a. Hospital standardization. *Surg. Gynec. Obstet.* 30: 641–647.

———. 1920b. The process of hospital standardization. *Surg. Gynec. Obstet.* 30: 543–544.

American Hospital Association. 1977. Hospital regulation. Report of the Special Committee on the Regulatory Process. Chicago: American Hospital Association.

American Jewish Congress and Community Action Resources for the Elderly. 1977. Patients and their complaints: a critical study of New York State's nursing home ombudsman—a joint report. Mimeographed. New York: American Jewish Congress and Community Action Resources for the Elderly.

Banta, D. 1979. Policies toward medical technology in developed countries. Paper read at the American Public Health Association meeting, 5 November, New York.

Berki, S. E. 1972. *Hospital economics.* Lexington, Mass.: Lexington Books.

Berliner, H. 1975. A larger perspective on the Flexner report. *Int. J. Health Serv.* 5: 573–590.

Bernstein, L. 1977. Personal communication.

Bicknell, R. 1977. Personal communication.

Brazda, J. F. 1979. Washington report: May, p. 3. *The Nation's Health.*

Butler, P. A. 1980. *Nursing Home Quality of Care Enforcement: Part I—Litigation by Private Parties, Part II—State Agency Enforcement Remedies.* Research Institute on Legal Services, Legal Services Corporation (limited circulation).

Cooper, B., and Worthington, N. 1973. National health expenditures 1929–72. *Soc. Sec. Bulletin.* 36: 3-19, 40.

Cooros, E. 1971. Rules hurt nursing homes. Rochester, N.Y. *Democrat and Chronicle.* 28 December.

Cristoffel, T. 1976. Medical care evaluation: an old new idea. *J. Med. Educ.* 51(2): 83–88.

Davis, L. 1960. *Fellowship of surgeons: a history of the American College of Surgeons.* Springfield, Ill.: Charles C. Thomas.

Demkovich, L. E. 1979. In treating the problems of the elderly, there may be no place like home. *Nat. J.* 22: 2154–58.

Dunlop, B. D. 1979. *The growth of nursing home care.* Lexington, Mass.: D. C. Heath.

Elliot, W. B. 1976. An investigtion of some effects of the New York State prospective reimbursement program on a group of upstate hospitals. Thesis, Cornell University.

Ellis, B. 1977. New JCAH president faces problems and opportunities. *Hospitals* 51: 92–96.

Ellwood, P. 1974. *Alternatives to regulation: improving the market.* Minneapolis: Interstudy.

Feder, J. M. 1977. *Medicare: the politics of federal hospital insurance.* Lexington, Mass.: D. C. Heath.

Feder, J. M. and Scanlon, W. 1980. Regulating the bed supply in nursing homes. *Milbank Memorial Fund Quarterly.* 58: 54–87.

Federation of State Medical Boards of the United States. 1979a. *Report of board actions for period 1973-1978.* Fort Worth, Texas: Federation of State Medical Boards of the United States.

———. 1979b. *Breakdown as to reasons for disciplinary actions taken by the boards and reported to FSMB 1973-1978.* Fort Worth, Texas: Federation of State Medical Boards of the United States.

Feld v. *Berger* 424 F. Supp. 1356. (S.D.N.Y., 1976).

Feldstein, P. J. 1979. *Health care economics.* New York: Wiley.

Freidman, M. 1962. *Capitalism and freedom.* Chicago: Univ. of Chicago Press.

Freidson, E. 1970. *Professional dominance: the social structure of medical care.* New York: Atherton.

———. 1975. *Doctoring together: a study of professional social control.* New York: Elsevier.

——— and Rhea, B. 1963. Process of control in a company of equals. *Soc. Prob.* 11(2): 119–131.

Fuchs, V. 1974. *Who shall live: health economics and social choice.* New York: Basic Books.

Galkin, F., and Sullivan, E. W. 1980. *Discharge planning in long-term facilities — no deposit, no return.* New York: Center for Policy Research, Inc. (limited circulation).

Ganey, T. 1978. Sikeston firm's nursing homes get more funds. *St. Louis Post-Dispatch.* 14 May, p. 1.

Gibson, R. M. 1979. National health expenditures, 1978. *Health Care Financing Rev.* 1: 1–36.

———. National health expenditures, 1979. *Health Care Financing Rev.* 2: 1–36.

Glanzman, B. 1978. Benefits of an ombudsman to a nursing home. Report on the nursing home patient ombudsman program, New York State Office of the Aging, unpublished paper.

Goldstein, T. 1976. The law is never far from public officials. *New York Times.* 18 April, p. 1, sec. 4.

Greenhouse, L. 1976. Albany adopts $10.78 billion budget. *New York Times.* 18 March, p. 45.

Grimaldi, P. L. 1980. Settling medicaid reimbursement rates for nursing home care: politics, procedure, and problems. South Orange, N.J.: Seton Hall University (Draft) June.

Havighurst, C. C. 1980. *Competition in a regulated health care system.* Washington, D.C.: Federal Trade Commission.

Hellinger, F. J. 1976. The effect of certificate of need legislation on hospital investment. *Inquiry* 13: 187–93.

———. 1979. *Cost benefit analysis of health care: past applications and future prospects.* Washington, D. C.: Office of Health Regulations, Health Care Financing Administration, Department of Health, Education, and Welfare.

Henderson, L. in Somers, H., and Somers, A. 1961. *Doctors, patients, and health insurance.* Washington, D.C.: Brookings Institution, p. 136.

Hess, J. 1975a. Stein clears Rockefeller of a nursing home taint. *New York Times.* 21 March, p. 22.

———. 1975b. Wilson says he saw Bergman twice on home but didn't do him favors. *New York Times.* 27 March, p. 60.

———. 1975c. Windfall indicated for nursing homes. *New York Times.* 23 May, p.1.

———. 1975d. Blumenthal calls charge 'outrageous, unfounded'. *New York Times.* 6 December, p.1., 40.

———. 1976. Bergman pleads guilty to a fraud in Medicaid and bribing Blumenthal. *New York Times.* 12 March, p.1.

Hospital Association of New York State. 1978. *Cost of regulation.* New York: Hospital Association of New York State.

Hospital Association of Pennsylvania. 1977. *The impact of government regulation on hospital costs.* Camp Hill, Pa.: Hospital Association of Pennsylvania.

Hynes, C. J. 1976. *Investigation into allegations of criminality in the nursing home industry in the state of New York.* First annual report to Governor Hugh L. Carey by the Special State Prosecutor. New York: Special State Prosecutor for Health and Social Services.

———. 1977. *Second annual report.* New York: Special State Prosecutor for Health and Social Services.

———. 1978a. *Third annual report.* Special State Prosecutor for Health and Social Services.

———. 1978b. The Willow Point Nursing Home and health related facility, prepared by L. N. Gray and J. Meekins. New York: Special State Prosecutor for Health and Social Services.

———. 1978c. Analysis of New York's profit-making long-term care facilities. New York: Special State Prosecutor for Health and Social Services.

———. 1979. *Fourth annual report.* New York: Special State Prosecutor for Health and Social Services.

Illich, I. 1976. *Medical nemesis.* New York: Pantheon.

Joint Commission on the Accreditation of Hospitals. 1979. Long-term care facilities accredited by the JCAH. Mimeographed. Chicago: Joint Commission on the Accreditation of Hospitals.

Johnson. D. 1977. JCAH plans stiffer, but not costlier, standards under new director Affeldt. *Mod. Health.* 7(9): 60–62.

Kahn, A. 1971. *The economics of regulation.* New York: Wiley.

Kaye, et al. v. *Whalen.* 405 N.Y.S.2d.632. 1978 App. Div.

Kessel, R. A. 1958. Price discrimination in medicine. *J. Law Econ.* 1: 20–53.

Kinzer, D. M. 1977. *Health controls out of control: warnings to the nation from Massachusetts.* Chicago: Teach 'Em.

Levine v. *Whalen,* 384 N.Y.S. 2d 721 (1976 App Div).

Little, A. D., Inc. 1975. *The long-term health care delivery system in New York State: issues and suggested approaches.* Report to the New York State Health Facilities Association. New York: Arthur D. Little Inc.

MacEachern, M. T. 1935. *Hospital organization and management.* Chicago: Physician's Record.

Maxwell v. *Wyman,* 458 f. 1146 (2d Cir. 1972).

McClure, W. 1978. *A comprehensive market and regulatory cost containment strategy for health care.* Unpublished manuscript.

McKinney's Session Law News of New York. 1976. St. Paul, Minn.: West.

Moreland Act Commission on Nursing Homes and Residential Facilities. 1975. *Regulating nursing home care: the paper tigers.* New York: Moreland Act Commission.

———. 1976a. *Reimbursement of nursing home property costs: pruning the money tree.* New York: Moreland Act Commission.

———. 1976b. *Political influence and political accountability: one foot in the door.* New York: Moreland Act Commission.

———. 1976c. *Reimbursing operating costs: dollars without sense.* New York: Moreland Act Commission.

———. 1976d. *Assessment and placement: anything goes.* New York: Moreland Act Commission.

———. 1976e. *Long term care regulation: past lapses, future prospects: a summary report.* New York: Moreland Act Commission.

Murawski, T. 1979. Unscrupulous physician. *New York Journal of Medicine:* 1021–28.

National Center for Health Statistics. 1980. Personal communication.

Newfield, J. 1975. Latest nursing home scandal: the Sigety cover-up. *Village Voice.* 13 January, p.14.

New York [Public Health] Law. Article 28.

New York State Department of Health. Board of Examiners of Nursing Home Administration. 1971–1978. *Annual report.* Albany.

———. Council's office. 1980a. Personal communication.

———. Division of Health Facilities Standards. 1977. *Program plan for residential health care facility surveillance.* Mimeographed copy, 6 May.

———. Division of Hospital Affairs. 1979a. *1966–1978, nursing home bed openings, by number of beds and region.* Mimeographed copy.

———. Division of Hospital Affairs. 1979b. *1966–1978 nursing home closings by home and region.* Mimeographed copy.

————. Office of Health Systems Management. 1977. *Status and implementation of chapter 900 of the laws of 1977; reporting of abuses of patients in residential health care facilities by professional and non-professional personnel.* Albany.

————. Office of Health Systems Management. 1978a. Computer printouts.

————. Office of Health Systems Management. 1978b. Transcripts of Flower City Nursing Home hearings, 30 March.

————. Office of Health Systems Management. 1978c. Personal communication.

————. Office of Health Systems Management. 1979a. *Nursing homes in New York State by region and latest rating as of 12-14-78.* Mimeographed copy.

————. Office of Health Systems Management. 1979b [1979c,d,e,]. *Patient abuse reporting statistical analysis.* Mimeographed copy, 15 April [31 July, 15 October, 31 December].

————. Office of Health Systems Management. 1979f. Personal communication.

————. Office of Health Systems Management. 1979g. *Second annual report to the governor and the legislature, chapter 900 requirements governing reporting of patient abuse in residential health care facilities.* Albany.

New York State Department of Social Service. Public Information Office. 1980 (January). Personal communication.

————. Office of the Special Prosecutor. 1980. Personal communication.

————. Program of Health Care Standards. 1976 [1977]. Health Facilities Directory: Nursing home. Albany: New York State Department of Health.

New York State Hospital code. 1976. Part 731.2(a)(1)(2).

New York Times. 1976. Hiring of auditors by Hynes opposed. 20 March, p. 17.

————. 1976b. Bergman license faces revocation. 13 March, p. 50.

————. 1974. (untitled). 13 August, p. 15.

O'Brannon v. *Town Court Nursing Center.* 586f.2d.280 (1979).

Owen, J. K. 1962. *Modern concepts of social administration.* Philadelphia: Saunders.

People of the State of New York v. *Albert Blumenthal* (1976 App Div), 55 2d 13.

Pirsig, R. M. 1974. *Zen and the art of motorcycle maintenance: an inquiry into values.* New York: William Morrow.

Posner, R. A. 1971. Taxation by regulation. *Bell J. Econ. Man. Sci. 2: 22–50.*

Prial, F. 1975. Report by Cuomo on nursing homes cites wide abuses. *New York Times.* 17 January, p.1, 30.

Program of Health Care Standards & Enforcement. 1976(1977). *Health facilities directory: nursing home.*

Public Law 90-248. 2 January 1968. *Social Security Amendments of 1967.* 81 Stat. 821.

Public Law 92-603. 30 October 1972. *Social Security Amendments of 1972.* 86 Stat. 1329.

Rayack, E. 1967. *Professional power and American medicine.* Cleveland: World.

Rensselaer Polytechnic Institute. 1979. *Regulation of long-term care in New York State phase I—system description.* Troy, N.Y.: Rensselaer Polytechnic Institute School of Management.

Rice, D. 1978. Projection and analysis of health status trends. Paper read at the American Public Health Association meeting in Washington, D.C. 17 October 1978.

Ruchlin, H. S., and Levey, S. 1972. Nursing home cost analysis: a case study. *Inquiry* 9: 3–15.

Salkever, D. S., and Bice, T. W. 1979. *Hospital certificate-of-need controls, impact of investments, cost, and use.* Washington, D. C.: American Enterprise Institute Studies in Health Policy.

Schlenker, R., and Graber, L. 1972. *Public utility regulation for the health care industry? Lessons from other regulated industries.* Minneapolis: Interstudy.

Schorr, B. 1978. FTC officer rules against AMA in care pivotal to health care antitrust effort. *Wall Street Journal.* 29 November, sec. 6, p. 59.

Schumacher, E. F. 1975. *Small is beautiful: economies as if people mattered.* New York: Harper & Row.

Shulman, D., and Galanter, R. 1976. Reorganizing the nursing home industry: a proposal. *Milbank Memorial Fund Quarterly.* 54(2): 129.

Slater, P. E. 1970. *Pursuit of loneliness: American culture at the breaking point.* Boston: Beacon.

Smith, D., and Kaluzny, A. 1975. *The white labyrinth.* Berkeley: McCutchan.

Solnick v. *Whalen.* 63A.D.2d.1062 (1978 App. Div.).

Somers, A. 1969. *Hospital regulation: the dilemma of public policy.* Princeton, N.J.: Princeton University Press Industrial Relations Section.

Spitz, B. 1979. *Medicaid nursing home reimbursement in New York.* Washington, D.C.: Urban Institute.

State of New York. Executive Budget. FY1965/6 to FY1978/9.

Sullivan, E. W. 1980. *Senior participation in corrective mechanisms.* New York: Center for Policy Research, Inc. (Mimeographed copy).

Temporary State Commission on Living Costs and the Economy. 1975. *Report on nursing homes and health related facilities in New York State.* New York: Temporary State Commission on Living Costs and the Economy.

Thomas, W. C., Jr. 1969. *Nursing homes and public policy: drift and decision in New York State.* New York: Cornell Univ. Press.

U.S. Congress. 1979. Introduction of legislation to halt federal trade commission restrictions on health care professionals. 96th Cong., 1st sess. *Cong. Rec.* 125: H1783 (28 March).

U.S. Congress, House of Representatives, Committee on Interstate and Foreign Commerce. 1977. Medicare-Medicaid antifraud and abuse amendments. Rep. No. 95-393, Part II. Washington, D.C.: Government Printing Office.

U.S. Congress, Senate, Committee on Finance. 1967. Social Security Amendment of 1967. 90th Cong., 1st sess., H.R. 12080, Part 2.

U.S. Congress, Senate, Committee on Government Affairs, Subcommittee on Federal Spending Practice and open Government. 1978. Assuring quality of care in nursing homes participating in Medicare and Medicaid. Washington, D.C.: Government Printing Office. (August) pp. 191–227.

U.S. Department of Health, Education, and Welfare. 1977a. Profile of chronic illness in nursing homes, United States: national nursing home survey, August 1973–April 1974. *Vital health statistics.* Ser. 13, No. 29. Washington, D.C.: Department of Health, Education, and Welfare.

———. 1977b. Characteristics, social contacts, and activities of nursing home residents, United States: 1973-1974 national nursing home survey. *Vital health statistics.* Ser. 13, No. 27. Washington, D.C.: Department of Health, Education, and Welfare.

University of Pittsburgh. 1959. *Hospital law manual.* Pittsburgh: Health Law Center.

Vladeck, B. 1980. *Unloving care.* New York: Basic Books.

Warner, G. M. 1979. Nursing home surveillance: what's wrong? Washington, D.C.: Health Facilities Standards and Control (Mimeographed copy).

Yaretsky v. *Blum* (DCNY, 1979). 456 F. Supp. 653.

Index

Abberman, Jan, 93
Abuse of patients
    attempts to control, 99, 112-13, 129,
        136-38, 142-43
    reporting of, 131-32, 135-40
Abzug, Bella, 145
Administration on Aging. See H.E.W.:
    Administration on Aging
American College of Physicians, 5
American College of Surgeons, 1-6, 18, 60
American Hospital Association, 5
AMA, 1-2, 5, 19, 35
Anderson, Warren, 116, 118
Article 28. See New York State Health
    Law, Article 28
Article 78. See New York State Health
    Law, Article 78

Bankruptcy of health care facilities, 38,
    77-78
Bergman, Bernard, 94, 108, 114, 116, 145
Blumenthal, Albert, 114, 115
Blue Cross, 5, 8n, 9, 60

Canadian Medical Association, 5
Carey, Hugh, 13-15, 95-96, 97
Carter, Rosalynn, 145
Certificates of Need
    consumer control, 147, 152
    in licensing health care facilities, 27-28
    in New York State, 60
    and patient care, 126, 134

Chill, Daniel C., 114
Clark, Ramsey, 145
Closure of health care facilities
    operator resistance to, 38-41
    the patient, 36-38, 149
    standards, 36-43, 84, 149
Council on Medical Education. See AMA:
    medical education
Consumer interests. See also Control
    mechanisms
    class action suits, 132, 141, 141-42
    early history of, 127-29, 133, 152-53
    government agencies as advocates for,
        138-40
    information for, 78, 84, 130
    ombudsman program, 141
    patients as, 127
    patient rights, 48, 129, 130-31, 134, 141,
        150, 152-53
    problems in, 129, 133-34, 146-47, 150
    regulation of the health care industry,
        46, 48-50, 113, 126-27, 127-28, 129,
        129-33, 133-34, 134-35, 142-43,
        150, 153-56
    success and failure of, 146, 150, 152-53
Consumer organizations
    1199, 135
    Caring Community, 145-46
    Coalition of Institutionalized Aged, 133
    Community Action Resources for the
        Elderly, 133, 134-135, 143
    Friends and Relatives of the Institu-
        tionalized Aged, 133, 134-35, 143

Grey Panthers, 135, 142-43
Legal Services for the Elderly Poor, 133, 134-35, 142-43, 145-46
New York State Association of Retired Persons, 128
New York State Charitable Aid Association, 143, 146-47
New York State Retired Teachers Association, 128
Continuing education. *See* Training
Control mechanisms. *See also* Government regulation
conflicts between, 53, 121, 128, 146-47
constituent and consumer, 127-29, 143, 146-47, 148, 150
criminal prosecution as, 150
general history of, 19-20, 122-25, 127-29, 148-49
ideals and assumptions in, 19-20, 52, 128
professional, 1-6, 19, 52, 91, 121, 127-28, 134, 148-49
public, 10, 121, 128, 146-47, 148
social utility of, 1, 127-28
voluntary, 5
Cost-based care rates, 60-65, 68, 69, 71-73
Cost control. *See* Management assessment
Council on Medical Education. *See* AMA
Criminal activities. *See also* Abuse; Fraud
attempts to control, 68, 70-72, 77-78, 86-87, 97-99, 150
bankruptcy, 77-78
kickbacks as, 99, 101-2
political corruption as, 13-14, 24, 65, 94-96, 99, 113-20
press coverage of, 94
prosecution of, 91-94, 99-102, 104, 106-8, 109, 111, 112-13, 150
Cuomo, Mario, 95-96, 113

Douglas, Robert, 114

Enforcement of regulations. *See also* Abuse; Criminal activities; Grievances
control mechanisms, 91, 121, 125, 149
current trends, 52-55, 149
as deterrent, 108-9, 120, 149, 150
disciplinary actions in, 29-33, 33-36, 36-43, 70, 84, 102, 149, 150
funding, 20-21, 97-99, 110-11

judicial intervention into, 35
New York State Health Department and, 24, 45, 70-71, 97-99, 106
New York State Special Prosecutor and, 15-16, 26, 29, 70-71, 91, 106, 113
by Nixon Administration, 22
problems in, 21-24, 33-35, 45-46, 52, 53-55, 84, 150
procedures for, 22-24, 29, 34-36, 76-77, 104
reforms in, 16-18, 25-26, 68, 78-79, 93, 106, 149

Federal Hospital Insurance Trust Fund, 72-73
Federal regulations and standards
Hill-Burton Act, 6, 20
Older Americans Act, Title III, 140, 140-41. *See also* Medicaid and Medicare; N.F.P.A. Life Safety Code; U.S. Social Security Act
state regulations, 20, 57, 78-79, 93
Title XVIII, 9, 70
Title XIX, 70
Financing patient care
cost-based reimbursement, 60-62
effects of public, 11, 60-61, 126
eligibility for, 7-8, 20-21, 57, 61
by federal agencies, 10-13, 46, 61
history of, 5, 13-16, 57
by New York State agencies, 10-13, 21, 60-61
recovery on fraud, 105-6
Fines. *See* Enforcement
Folsom, Marion B., 9, 60
Fraud. *See also* New York State Civil Recovery Unit; Recovery
as criminal activity, 13-14, 62-65, 66, 68-69, 86-87, 93, 99-101, 102, 104, 109, 118, 129, 150
in Medicare and Medicaid, 74, 86-88, 99, 101-2, 104, 104-5

Government regulation, xiv
Grievances by patients, 127, 131, 135, 146-47. *See also* Abuse; Ombudsman

H.E.W.
Administration on Aging, 131
enforcement of regulatory standards, 22, 23

funding by, 21, 76, 131
licensing of health care facilities, 8-10
reviews of local operations, 8, 21, 109
Hill-Burton Act. *See* Federal regulations
    and standards
Hollander, Eugene, 108
Hurd, T. Norman, 114
Hynes, Charles, 94, 96, 108-9, 115, 116

Ingraham, Hollis, 15
Inspections and audits of health care
        facilities. *See also* Ombudsman
    changes resulting from, 66, 149
    costs of, 21, 21n, 65, 97-99
    cost control, 44
    current problems in, 43, 53-55, 106, 151
    by government agencies, 8, 10, 33, 128
    in the nineteenth century, 57, 127
    Periodic Medical Reviews, 33, 50
    posting results of, 130, 133-34
    procedures and staffing of, 22, 26-27,
        33-34, 49-50, 59, 66, 97
    response of Nursing Home Association
        to, 65
Inspectors
    recruited from F.B.I. and police
        departments, 97
    operators of health care facilities, 11-13,
        16, 21, 24, 26, 41-43, 80, 81, 93, 99,
        121, 133, 138-40, 152-53
    centralized investigators, 26-27, 121
Interagency conflicts
    federal vs. state agencies, 8-10, 20-21,
        53, 78-79, 128
    in New York State, 20, 24, 27, 48, 53,
        73, 102, 106, 109, 109-12, 116,
        117-18, 120, 122
Interagency cooperation
    federal vs. state agencies, 20, 21, 57,
        97-99, 106, 109, 140, 140-41
    in New York State, 59

Joint Commission for Accreditation of
        Hospitals (J.C.A.H.)
    as a control mechanism, 19, 149
    costs of health care, 11, 60
    the courts, 35
    federal funding of health care, 10
    founding of, 5
    licensing health care staff, 52

licensing hospitals, 8-10
vs. Social Security Administration, 8

Kaplan, Louis I., 91-92, 93
Koch, Edward, 145

Lefkowitz, Lewis, 94, 114
Legislative ethics bill, 140
Liability of operators, 67-68, 132
Licensing of health care facilities
    Codman Report on, 2-4
    conflicts between agencies in, 8-10
    criteria for, 26, 27-28, 28-33, 45-46,
        60, 61, 76-78
    as enforcement procedure, 113, 149
    the federal government and, 8-10, 28
    fiscal criteria for, 45-46, 61, 76-77,
        77-78
    history of, 28-29
    as hospitals, 6-8, 9, 10, 28
    by J.C.A.H., 5, 8-10
    by New York State agencies, 20, 26-29,
        61, 69, 128
    as nursing homes, 5-6, 9, 10, 20, 26, 28
Licensing of physicians and medical schools
    Federation of State Medical Boards
        report on, 29-32
    general, 1-2
    Carnegie Foundation and, 2
    Flexner Report and, 2
    patient abuse reporting, 136, 138
    by professional organizations, 1-6
    Rockefeller Foundation and, 2
Life Safety Code. *See* N.F.P.A. Life Safety
    Code
Lombardi, Tarki, 16
Lowell, Stanley, 114

Management assessments
    in conflict with regulatory standards,
        43-46, 76-77, 150
    effects and results of, 45-46, 60-61,
        77-78, 150
    emphasized, 44, 149
    by New York State agencies and codes,
        45, 61, 76-77
    licensing of health care facilities, 77-78
    problems with, 45
    required by courts, 76
    vs. social work, 44-45

Management of health care facilities, 151

Marchi, John, 114

Medicaid and Medicare
costs of health care, 10-11, 57, 61, 62,
68-69, 71-73, 74-77, 78, 149
the courts, 35, 106-8
the Federal Hospital Insurance Trust
Fund, 72-73
Fraud Abuse Bill of 1977, 97-99
licensing and certification of health care
facilities, 7-10, 19, 20, 33
patient compared to private payment
patients, 126
proprietary nursing home reimbursement, 86
regulatory standards, 9, 10-13, 20,
21-22, 35, 60, 66, 93, 132-33,
146-50
requirements and criteria for, 7-8, 10,
20, 61
state agencies, 106

Medical schools. *See* Licensing of
physicians and medical schools

Melia, Aloysius J., 114

National Advisory Council on Nursing
Home Administrators, 28

New York City agencies and codes
Commission on Welfare, 59
Community Council of Greater New
York City, 140-41
Department of Investigations, 59, 91-92,
93
Heyman Commission Report, 59
Nursing Home Code, 59

New York State agencies and codes
Assembly Subcommittee on Health
Care Reform, 16-18
Board of Examiners of Nursing Home
Administrators, 26, 28-29, 33
Bureau of Audits and Investigators, 66,
104-6, 110-12
Bureau of Health Economics, 21
Bureau of Residential Health Care
Reimbursement, 66
Charities Relief Association, 57
Civil Recovery Unit, 106-8
Code Title X, 131
Committee on Hospital Costs, 60
Department of Social Services, 20, 106,
141

Division of Audit Appeals, 104-5
Division of Budget, 45, 65, 77, 78, 135
Division of Health Economics, 62, 118
Division of Health Facilities Standards,
43
Division of Long-term Care Reimburse-
ment, 45
Governor's Committee on Hospital
Costs, 9
Health Care Financing Administration
Division of Long-term Care, 46
Hospital Review and Planning Council,
10
Joint Legislative Task Force on Resi-
dential Health Care Facilities, 72-73
Medicaid Program, 10, 21, 78, 94-96,
150
Metcalf-McCloskey Act, 60
Moreland Act Commission, 15-16,
24-26, 45, 64-65, 68-69, 72-73,
86-87, 113-14, 116, 120, 130, 140
Nursing Home Code, 41, 46
Office for the Aging, 131, 136, 140-41,
147
Office of Health Systems Management,
10, 21, 44, 66, 84, 110, 138
Office of Nursing Home Affairs, 22
Office of Public Health, 66
Office of the Special Prosecutor, 15, 26,
48, 70-71, 74, 87, 91, 96, 97-99,
99-102, 104-5, 106-12, 112-13,
115-20, 121-25, 131, 135, 136-38,
143, 146
Old Age Securities Act of 1930, 57
Public Health Council, 65, 71, 73
Public Health Law Article 28, 9, 10, 20,
28-29, 36, 60, 61, 74, 93
Public Health Law Article 78, 76, 104,
111
Public Health Law Amendments, 36,
135-38
Public Welfare Law of 1929, 127-28
Task Force on the Nursing Home Code,
46-50
Temporary Commission on Living Costs
and the Economy, 13-16, 24, 62-64,
68-69, 92, 93-94, 114, 116

N.F.P.A. Life Safety Code, 22, 36, 52, 53,
74, 128, 145-46

Nurses, 60, 79, 141. *See also* Abuse

Ombudsman, 93, 131, 140-41, 147
Operators of health care facilities
  continuing education for, 29
  as criminals, 99, 109
  firing employees for patient abuse, 113
  ombudsman program, 140, 141
  rating of health care facilities, 82-84,
    133
  reform, 70, 136
  See also Inspectors
Ownership of health care facilities, 74,
  132-33, 142-46, 146-47

Patient Care
  availability, 37-38, 72, 74, 126-27, 149
  costs. *See also* Management assessments
    government funding or reimbursement,
      11, 46, 60-62, 64, 126
    inflation of, 11-12, 48-49, 53, 60, 64
    in nursing homes compared to other
      health care facilities, 60-61, 64
    present trends, 11, 64
    public concern over, 57
    related to quality of care, 43-46, 53,
      64
    reviewed by regulatory bodies, 9, 10,
      24, 46, 64-65
  quality
    costs related to, 43-46, 53
    effects of government funding on, 46,
      79-80
    incentives to improve, 70, 85-86
    linked to reimbursement rates, 45-46,
      69-70, 71, 73-74, 79-80, 84, 87-88
    monitoring of, 85, 131
    New York State agencies, regulation
      of, 10, 11, 24, 46, 73-74
    and ombudsman, 141
    professional controls on, 4-6, 134
    in proprietary nursing homes, 86
    rating of, 69
    reform of, 126-29, 134-35
    See also Inspections of health care
      facilities; Licensing of health care
      facilities; Consumer interests
Patient Bill of Rights. *See* Consumer
  interests
Periodic Medical Review. *See* Inspection of
  health care facilities
Physicians, 5, 126, 136-38, 141. *See also*
  Licensing of physicians

Political corruption. *See* Criminal activities
Press coverage of health care
  coverage and health care industry, 24,
    94, 128-29, 130, 133, 143, 146
  John Hess and *New York Times,* 13, 69,
    94
  Jack Newfield of *Village Voice,* 13, 94
  regulators use of, 133
Proprietary nursing homes
  bankruptcy of, 77-78, 144-45
  collaborative efforts in New York City,
    59
  consumer pressure, 126-27, 132-33
  defection of regulatory agency staff to,
    88
  effects of capital-cost reimbursement on,
    73, 74, 76-77, 79-80
  emergence of, 57, 128, 132-33
  fraud in, 87, 109
  Medicaid, 86
  Moreland Act Commission on, 86-87
  as political issue, 133
  quality of care in, 84, 91-92
  regulation of, 59, 61
  reimbursement, 86-87
  related to voluntary nursing homes, 69,
    74, 76-77, 79-80, 86-87, 109, 119,
    140, 144-45
Proprietary Nursing Home Organization.
  See Trade associations
Public Health Council, 33-34
Public Health Service, 9

Rating quality in health care facilities.
  See also Reimbursement; Patient
    care quality; Standards; Inspections
  calculation of, 80-81, 85, 85-87, 133,
    134
  consumer interests, 130, 133, 133-34,
    150
  fiscal controls, 85-87
  flaws in, 81-83, 150
  as incentive to improvement, 83-84
  Health Department codes, 70, 84
  problems with, 80, 82-84, 133, 134
  reimbursement, 80, 82-84, 84-90, 150
  appeal of, 82
Recovery against fraud, 93, 104-11
Reform in the nursing home industry
  compared between proprietary and
    voluntary homes, 79-80

concerning surveillance procedures,
49–50, 149
conflicting objectives in, 53, 80
consumer interest, 78, 130–31, 134–35,
136, 142–43, 146, 150
to control abuses, 71–72
effects of, 72–74, 79–80, 93, 126–29,
146, 150
fiscal, 53, 68, 68–69, 70–71, 73–74, 76,
77, 79–80
history of, 57, 60, 66–68, 73–74, 92,
122, 148–49
by government agency, 15–18, 25–26,
49–52, 66–68, 68–69, 70, 72, 113,
130–31
professional controls, 18, 50, 77, 148,
149
response of health care industry to, 16,
49–50, 76–77
Rehabilitative services, 60
Reimbursement
abuse of, 65, 69, 71–72
calculation of, 72–74, 76–77, 86–87
charge-based, 59–60
compared between nursing homes and
hospitals, 61–62
compared between voluntary and
proprietary nursing homes, 74,
76–77, 86–87, 119, 149
controls on, 69, 88, 118–20
cost-based, 59–60, 60–61, 62–64, 68
costs excluded from, 132, 141
criteria and certification for, 45–46,
62–64, 68, 70, 71–72, 78–80
effects of government funding of, 60–61,
68–69, 74–77
federal agencies, 56, 68–69, 70, 72–73,
74–77, 81, 118, 149
the health care system, 56, 149
as incentive to improvement, 70, 83–84,
91
labor relations, 88
linked to quality rating, 69–70, 71–72,
73–74, 77, 79–80, 81–82, 82–84,
84–90, 157
New York State agencies, 45, 60, 62–65,
66, 68–69, 71–72, 73–74, 77–78, 81,
84
New York State as model for, 62–64
nursing home trade associations, 72, 74,
76–77

political influence, 88
problems with, 56, 60–61, 62–65, 69, 74,
78–79, 80, 84–86
procedures for, 45, 60–61, 69
public confidence in, 73
reform of, 69, 70, 72–73, 73–74, 76,
78, 79–80, 84
rise in health care costs, 64–65
standards enforcement, 78–79, 84, 104,
149
of voluntary community group owners,
73
Rockefeller, Nelson, 9, 60, 93, 114

Sigety, Charles, 94
Stein, Andrew, 15, 113–14, 116, 130
Steingut, Stanley, 16, 94, 114, 116
Social issues
control of health services, 1, 127–28
vs. administrative efficiencies, 44–45
Social Security. *See* U.S. Social Security Act
Standards for regulating health care
bureaucratization of, 35–36, 91,
122–25, 148
compared between nursing homes and
hospitals, 10
conflicts in, 5, 44–45, 81
consumer interests as, 128, 134, 135,
146, 150
cost-control and, 35, 43–46, 53, 85, 150
cost reimbursement, 60–61, 78–79,
79–80
the courts and, 35–37, 152–53
current trends in, 36, 52–55, 149, 150
certification of compliance with, 45–46
Federal acts and agencies, 6–7, 60,
132–33
federal funding of health care, 7–8,
10–13
history of public, 5, 6–10, 60–61,
122–25, 129, 148–49
loss of profit, 61
mini/maxi, 48–49, 135
of New York State agencies, 6, 9, 10,
16–18, 46–50, 59, 60, 66, 81, 113,
131, 134–35
New York State consolidation of, 9
New York State objectives in, 93–94
the N.F.P.A. Life Safety Code, 22
as a political issue, 121–25, 151–52

professional controls and, 1-6, 8-10, 35-37, 50, 91, 148, 149
suggestion, for reform, 150-51
U.S. Social Security Act, 6-7
Surveillance. *See* Enforcement; Inspections; Standards regulation

Tanner, Marian, 145
Temporary Commission on Living Costs and the Economy. *See* New York State Temporary Commission on Living Costs and the Economy
Trade Associations
lobbying by, 49, 134-35
Metropolitan Nursing Home Association, 59
New York State Nursing Home Association, 16, 65
New York Association of Homes for the Aged, 76-77
New York State Proprietary Nursing Home Organization, 16
New York Health Care Facilities Association, 72, 74

Training
early history of, 60
costs, 59
of Health Department Staff, 50, 138
for nursing home staff, 28-29, 33, 113
of volunteer ombudsman staff, 140-41
Transfer of patients, 141, 142-43. *See also* Patient care

U.S. Senate Committee on Aging, 28
U.S. Health Quality and Standards Bureau, 46
U.S. Social Security Act
amendments to, 6-7, 28
nursing home licensing, 8-10, 28
based on New York State Old Age Securities Act of 1930, 57
public policy, 57
public regulation of health care, 6-7
cost of health care, 11

Wagner, Robert F., 91-92
Waife, Mitchell, 145
Warner, George, 46
Whalen, Robert, 15, 16, 78

About the Author

David Barton Smith is a Professor in the Department of Health Administration, which he also chairs, at Temple University in Philadelphia. He has served as Assistant Professor in the Sloan Program of Hospital and Health Services Administration within the Graduate School of Business and Public Administration at Cornell University, and as Visiting Assistant Professor in the Department of Preventive Medicine and Community Health in the School of Medicine and Dentistry at The University of Rochester. Dr. Smith is the co-author of two other books: THE WHITE LABYRINTH: UNDERSTANDING THE ORGANIZATION OF HEALTH CARE with A. Kaluzny, and CAREERS IN HEALTH with B. Zimmerman. Additionally, he has contributed to the journals *Medical Care, Inquiry, Social Science & Medicine,* and *Health Administration,* among others. He holds a Master of Arts degree in Social Science from Michigan State University and a Ph.D. in Medical Care Organization from the University of Michigan.